The Endocrine System

The Endocrine System

Miraculous Messengers

TORSTAR BOOKS
New York • Toronto

TORSTAR BOOKS INC.
300 E. 42nd Street,
New York, New York 10017

THE HUMAN BODY
The Endocrine System:
Miraculous Messengers

Publisher
Bruce Marshall

Art Director
John Bigg

Creation Coordinator
Harold Bull

Editor
John Clark

Managing Editor
Ruth Binney

Commissioning Editor
Hal Robinson

Contributors
Arthur Boylston, Julian Chomet,
Robert Goldin, Paulette Pratt, Saffron
Whitehead

Text Editors
Wendy Allen, Mike Darton, Martyn
Page, Sandy Shepherd

Researchers
Maria Pal, Jazz Wilson

Picture Researchers
Jan Croot, Kate Duffy, Dee Robinson

Layout and Visualization
Eric Drewery, Ted McCausland

Artists
Mick Gillah, Aziz Khan, Mick
Saunders, Shirley Willis

Cover Design
Moonink Communications

Cover Art
Paul Giovanopoulos

Production Director
Barry Baker

Production Coordinator
Janice Storr

Business Coordinator
Candy Lee

Planning Assistant
Avril Essery

International Sales
Barbara Anderson

In conjunction with this series
Torstar Books offers an electronic
digital thermometer which provides accurate body temperature
readings in large liquid crystal
numbers within 60 seconds.

For more information write to:
Torstar Books Inc.
300 E. 42nd Street
New York, NY 10017

Marshall Editions, an editorial group that
specializes in the design and publication of
scientific subjects for the general reader,
prepared this book. Marshall has written and
illustrated standard works on technology,
animal behavior, computer usage and the
tropical rain forests which are recommended
for schools and libraries as well as for
popular reference.

Series Consultants
Donald M. Engelman is Professor of
Molecular Biophysics and Biochemistry and
Professor of Biology at Yale. He has
pioneered new methods for understanding
cell membranes and ribosomes, and has also
worked on the problem of atherosclerosis.
He has published widely in professional and
lay journals and lectured at many
universities and international conferences.
He is also involved with National Advisory
Groups concerned with Molecular Biology,
Cancer, and the operation of National
Laboratory Facilities.

Stanley Joel Reiser is Professor of
Humanities and Technology in Health Care
at the University of Texas Health Science
Center in Houston. He is the author of
Medicine and the Reign of Technology; coeditor
of *Ethics in Medicine: Historical Perspectives and
Contemporary Concerns*; and coeditor of the
anthology *The Machine at the Bedside*.

Harold C. Slavkin, Professor of
Biochemistry at the University of Southern
California, directs the Graduate Program in
Craniofacial Biology and also serves as Chief
of the Laboratory for Developmental Biology
in the University's Gerontology Center. His

research on the genetic basis of congenital
defects of the head and neck has been
widely published.

Lewis Thomas is Chancellor of the Memorial
Sloan-Kettering Cancer Center in New York
City and University Professor at the State
University of New York, Stony Brook. A
member of the National Academy of
Sciences, Dr. Thomas has served on advisory
councils of the National Institutes of Health.

Consultants for The Endocrine
System
Barry J. Klyde is an Assistant Professor in
the Endocrinology Division of the
Department of Medicine at Cornell
University Medical College and an Assistant
Attending Physician at The New York
Hospital. He has conducted research into
endocrinology and metabolism and has
coauthored articles on these and related
topics.

Victor Schneider is an Associate Professor in
the Division of Endocrinology at the
University of Texas Medical School in
Houston. He is also Visiting Scientist at the
NASA-Johnson Space Center Medical
Research Branch in Houston, and Medical
Staff Officer at the National Institutes of
Health, Bethesda, Maryland. He is author or
coauthor of numerous articles on various
aspects of endocrinology, particularly with
regard to calcium metabolism in humans.

Terry Taylor is an Assistant Professor of
Medicine at Georgetown University
Hospital, Washington, DC, where she
teaches and practices endocrinology. She
also carries out experimental research in the

field of neuroendocrinology at the National
Institutes of Health in Bethesda. Many of her
recent publications have concerned the
functioning of the thyroid gland.

Medical Advisor
Arthur Boylston

© Torstar Books Inc. 1985

**Library of Congress
Cataloging in Publication Data**

Main entry under title:

The Endocrine System: Miraculous
Messengers.

Includes index.
1. Endocrine glands. 2. Endocrinology–
popular works. 3. Hormones–physiological
effect.
[DNLM: 1. Endocrine glands–physiology–
popular works. 2. Hormone–physiology–
popular works. WK 102 E556]
QP187.E55 1985 612'.4 85-21019

ISBN 0-920269-22-2 (The Human Body Series)
ISBN 0-920269-59-1 (The Endocrine System)
ISBN 0-920269-60-5 (leatherbound)
ISBN 0-920269-61-3 (school ed.)

20 19 18 17 16 15 14 13 12 11
10 9 8 7 6 5 4 3 2 1

Printed in Belgium

Contents

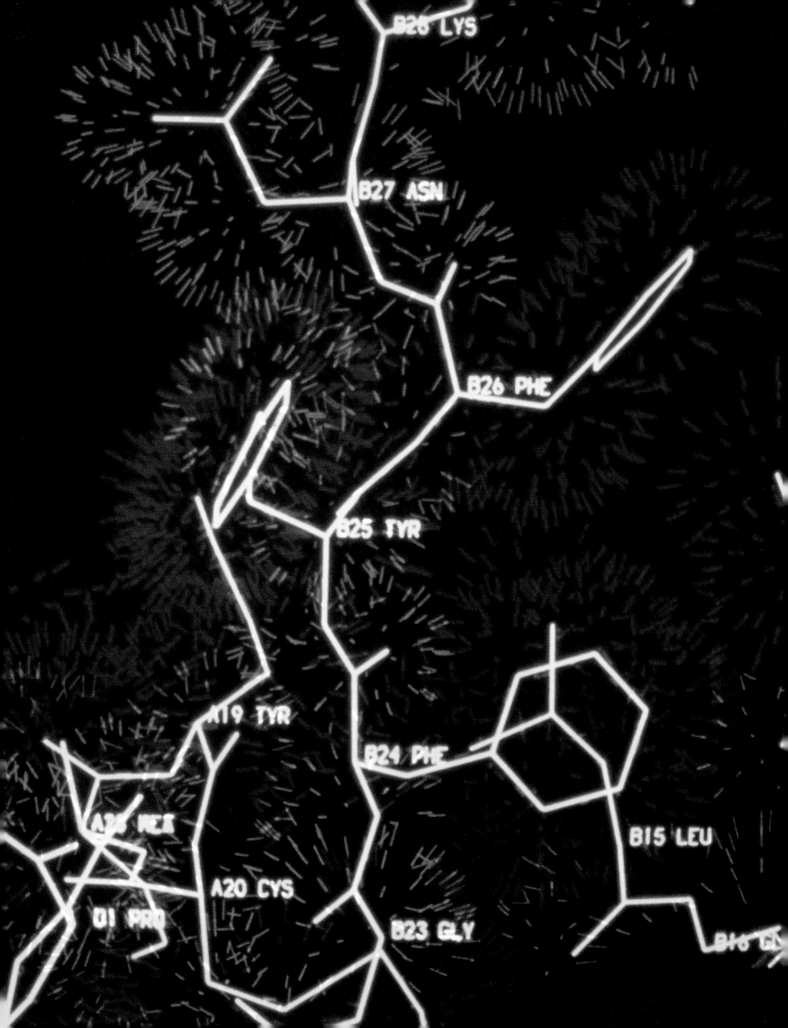

Introduction:

From Humors to Hormones

If you are said to be out of humor what is meant is that you are not your usual self, sunny or grouchy. The expression harks back to the ancient Greek notion of the four humors, the four body fluids (blood, phlegm, bile and choler), which as a theory achieved considerable popularity again in Medieval Europe. Then it was common for people to categorize others as "sanguine" (from the Latin for "blood"), "phlegmatic", "bilious" or "choleric," corresponding to what was judged to be the dominant humor in each. The terms are still used to denote dispositions (although some of them have changed their meanings somewhat).

It is interesting that in all traditions regarding humors, a central necessity is balance. If the correct balance in the body is maintained, one's life and disposition should be normal and well-adjusted; if there is a preponderance of one or another humor, however, the result is either a morbid characteristic or an illness.

The four humors as scientific realities have of course long been discarded. Certainly blood, bronchial mucus (phlegm) and gall (bile) are essential to the well-being of the body — but the substances now known to be as vital, and in the same sort of way as the humors were once supposed to be, are the hormones. These too require a critical balance for the maintenance of body systems, a balance that is constantly monitored and regulated by hormonal negative feedback. Reduction or excess of any hormones can lead to serious disorders at any time of life, starting from well before birth, as can any malfunction of the glands that produce them.

Endocrinology is one of the most exciting disciplines within modern biology; it has produced many useful advances, such as the synthesis of hormones, methods of contraception and combating infertility, and the treatment of disorders such as diabetes — once fatal, now easily and comfortably controllable.

A better understanding of the ways hormones work – and sometimes fail to work – comes from a knowledge of their molecular shape and structure. This complex analysis has been revolutionized in recent years by the use of computers, which not only sift and correlate a mass of physical and chemical data but also visualize the molecules as vivid computer graphics.

7

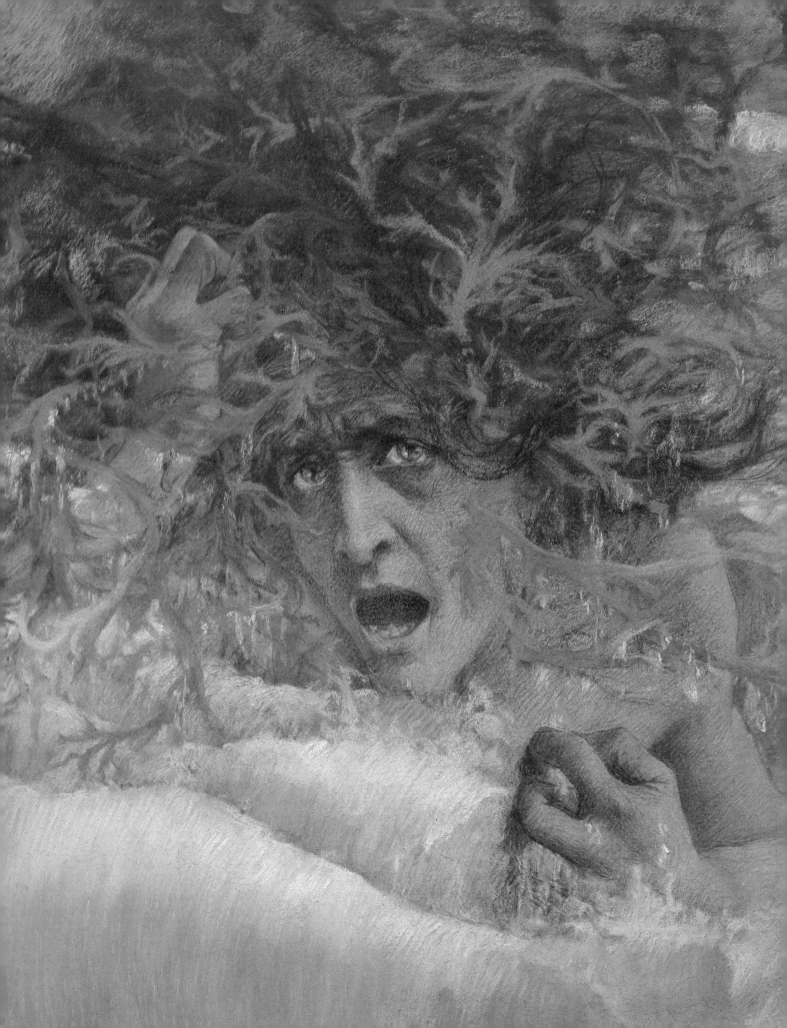

Chapter 1

History of Hormones

The human body uses subtle and complex communications systems to survive. Good internal communication within the body allows each of us to fight or flee, to eat and digest, to grow and develop, and to reproduce.

The more sophisticated a living organism is, the more important such communication becomes. In humans, the nervous system provides a high-speed transmission system utilizing electrochemical signals just like a giant computerized telephone network. The body also has a somewhat slower channel of internal communications, through a "canal" system — the bloodstream. The Englishman William Harvey established a monumental landmark in the history of medicine at the beginning of the seventeenth century, when he showed that blood circulated through the blood vessels, but another 250 years passed before it was realized that every organ of the body sends "messages" via the bloodstream to other organs and tissues.

In some ways the body's communication networks are comparable to the canal-linked city of Venice. A telephone call can deliver a message practically instantaneously, just like a nerve transmission. But a slower message can be sent by using a fleet of gondolas through the canals of Venice — one of them will reach any specific destination in the city, just like a chemical message that is sent in the blood.

As scientists unraveled the mysteries of the body's complex communications systems, they discovered that the most important of the organs that produced chemical messengers were small glandular structures under the control of complex regulatory mechanisms. The chemical messengers passed into the bloodstream from these glands are called hormones. Understanding of their precise roles had not begun until the middle of the nineteenth century, although anatomists did know about the glands responsible, known as ductless or

Hormones produced by the endocrine system can have a profound effect on physical appearance—although not so extreme as to turn a person into a snake-haired Medusa. Nevertheless, the effects can be dramatic; for example, an excess of pituitary growth hormone can result in gigantism, and an insufficiency of hormones from the adrenal cortex (which occurs in Addison's disease) causes, among other symptoms, bronzing of the skin.

9

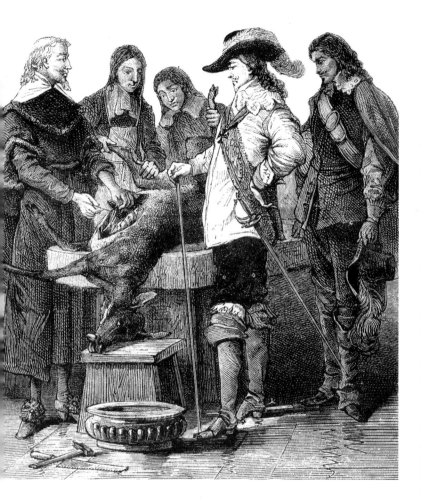

endocrine glands because they release their products directly into the bloodstream, not via a tube or duct.

In the 1930s, the whole endocrine process, with its regulatory mechanisms, was described as an orchestra. The glands discharging their products into the blood represented the playing musicians, while the conductor of the orchestra was the pituitary gland, which lies at the base of the brain. It is now known that hormones are vital to our health and well-being; if our glands work improperly we can become ill, even extremely so. Such knowledge is the result of hundreds of years of investigations in the field of endocrinology — the study of hormones and their effects — although mostly acquired since the 1950s.

The Beginnings of Endocrinology

In prehistoric times, organs such as the heart, gonads or brain were taken from slaughtered animals or human enemies and eaten in the belief that they would improve the consumer's health or confer the dead person's attributes and talents. Eating the heart of an enemy to obtain his bravery is now considered an act of cannibalism, but could

also be regarded as a crude form of "organo-therapy." The ancient Chinese developed remedies which included toad's skin for dropsy and hen's gizzard to treat indigestion and gastric ulcers.

Such practices may be said to be reflected in modern medicine in treatments for deficiencies due to the failure of certain endocrine organs to produce sufficient amounts of hormones. Treatments may take the form of injections of an extract made from a similar but healthy organ. Infertility was of great concern to the ancient Chinese, and the Egyptians are thought to have been just as concerned about contraception, even before 1000 B.C. They understood enough about endocrine and reproductive functions to have performed operations to remove ovaries for this very purpose.

Along with the Chinese and the Egyptians, the ancient Greeks also sought to cure the swelling in the thyroid gland at the front of the neck known as a goiter. The Greeks were correct in attributing the condition to the type of water drunk, and we now know that a lack of iodine in the diet predisposes to the formation of goiters.

In the Mediterranean world it was not only physicians who studied and practiced medicine but also priests, philosophers and gymnasts. Empedocles of Sicily (490–430 B.C.), a nomadic philosopher, physician and poet, popularized the contemporarily prevalent idea of the fourfold root of health: air, earth, fire and water. A little earlier, Pythagoras of Samos, famous for his mathematical theorem, had decided that these four elements should be related to four qualities: dry, moist, hot and cold. This, contended Pythagoras, produced the four humors of the body: blood, phlegm, yellow bile and black bile. Pythagoras went on to conclude that combinations and permutations of these three quartets of conditions explained disease and the action of drugs.

It was Hippocrates (460–370 B.C.), often called the father of medicine, who changed the face of the science of medicine from a mainly surgical one with applications only in war, to one that included internal medicine, physiology and pathology. He bravely rejected the idea that disease was caused by the intervention of gods and demons, and instead studied patients thoroughly, noting their general and overall condition: the face, temperature,

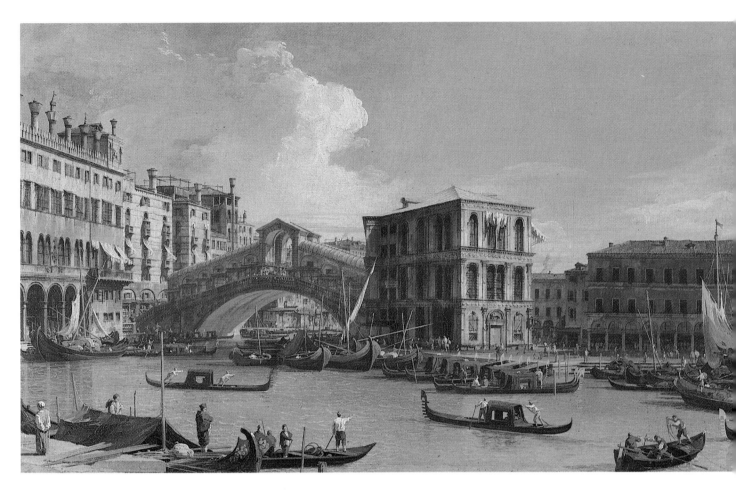

One of the many landmarks of Venice is the famous Rialto Bridge over the Grand Canal, depicted here by the city's equally renowned eighteenth-century artist Canaletto. Like the gondolas and other craft that still ply the maze of Venice's canal system, hormones secreted by the various endocrine glands travel through the body's network of blood vessels, producing effects far from their sites of production.

respiration, pulse and ease of body movement. From his observations he concluded that the four humors had to be correctly balanced in the body for good health. He was indeed correct in perceiving that a balance of substances in the body is necessary — but was somewhat misguided in believing that the right testicle produced male offspring and the left female.

Another remarkable Greek was Aristotle (348–322 B.C.), who was also interested in reproduction. He described the effect of castration in male birds with incredible accuracy, and compared their loss of fertility and male sexual characteristics with those of castrated men. Erroneously, though, he thought that the testes were merely weights responsible for tensioning the spermatic cords. His means of testing for fertility was to see whether a man's semen floated in water — if it did it was not fertile, but if it sank it was normal.

Yet another Greek, the greatest medical man of antiquity after Hippocrates, was Galen (A.D. 130–200). Son of an architect, he became the founder of experimental physiology, and much of his work had an enormous influence on medical

11

practice and opinion throughout the Middle Ages and up to the seventeenth century. He was without doubt the most skilled physician of the Greco-Roman period, although he did not have the high ethical standards of Hippocrates, nor his lucidity and honesty of experimental style. All the same he worked out and understood the actions of a number of drugs, including opium, and the effects and uses of turpentine, wine, honey, barley water and many other substances.

Galen's prominent status in endocrinological history derives from his anatomical isolation of the thyroid, pineal and pituitary glands. He thought, though, that the pituitary gland was responsible for passing the waste products of chemical reactions in the brain out through the nose as mucus. The thyroid gland he incorrectly described as secreting a fluid that lubricated the larynx.

The Renaissance

After the Greco-Roman period, the wheel of medical progress turned slowly indeed. Even at the start of the sixteenth century Aristotle was still regarded as the foremost teacher of medicine and biology. Galen remained the master of medicine: his books on anatomy were still being used to teach medical students. One man who disagreed with both these distinguished Greeks, however, was the swashbuckling Swiss physician Paracelsus, who publicly burned the works of Aristotle and Galen (although he had a little more respect for Hippocrates). He rejected traditional medicine, an attitude which made him many enemies. Some of his observations, however — such as the realization of a connection between cretinism, endemic goiters, and congenital idiocy (all caused by a deficiency of thyroid hormone) — assured him a deserved place in medical history. He also introduced a number of new drugs into the pharmacist's dispensary, such as iron compounds, arsenic, copper sulfate, mercury (particularly for treating syphilis), and potassium sulfate.

Other keen observers during the Renaissance were great artists, such as Leonardo da Vinci, who believed that true knowledge of anatomy could be acquired only by dissection. Da Vinci made more than 750 sketches of muscles, hearts, lungs, blood vessels and cross-sections of the brain. The founder of cross-sectional anatomy, he undoubtedly laid the foundations for modern medical anatomical drawings and paved the way toward a better understanding of the structure of glands.

Another excellent dissector was Andreas Vesalius (1514–1564), now described as the pioneer of modern anatomy. Part of what he taught students was to dissect and inspect the human organs within the body. Vesalius' main pupil, Gabriele Falloppio, later carried on Vesalius' superb anatomical work and provided a clearer picture of the glands within the body. Falloppio was to be immortalized through his discovery in 1561 of the Fallopian tubes, which connect the ovaries to the uterus.

Progress Toward Modern Endocrinology

It was not until the advent of the microscope in the seventeenth century that the detailed structure of the glands, so brilliantly isolated during the previous 150 years, could be studied. The female "organs of procreation" were studied by Reinier de Graaf and many others who utilized the new microscopes, although these instruments were only simple lenses in those early days. De Graaf, who was born in Holland, made a name for himself in endocrinological history by his discovery of how a (Graafian) follicle matures in the ovary, releases the ovum, or egg, and is later discarded. He was also one of the first to study the pancreas and its function, and he disproved the theory that the pancreas was the excretory organ of the spleen, analogous to the function of the gall bladder (which stores bile) in relation to the liver. De Graaf also made revolutionary observations on the structure of the testicles, noting that they consisted largely of tubules, known today as seminiferous tubules. What made the work of de Graaf even more remarkable is that he lived only to the age of 32, dying of unknown causes and thus tragically depriving the scientific world of a genius also known for his clarity, elegance and good humor.

One contemporary of de Graaf was the Englishman Thomas Willis, who teamed up with his pupil Richard Lower, to produce some of the most outstanding work of his generation. Willis was interested mainly in neurology, a field now known to be delicately interwoven with endocrinology,

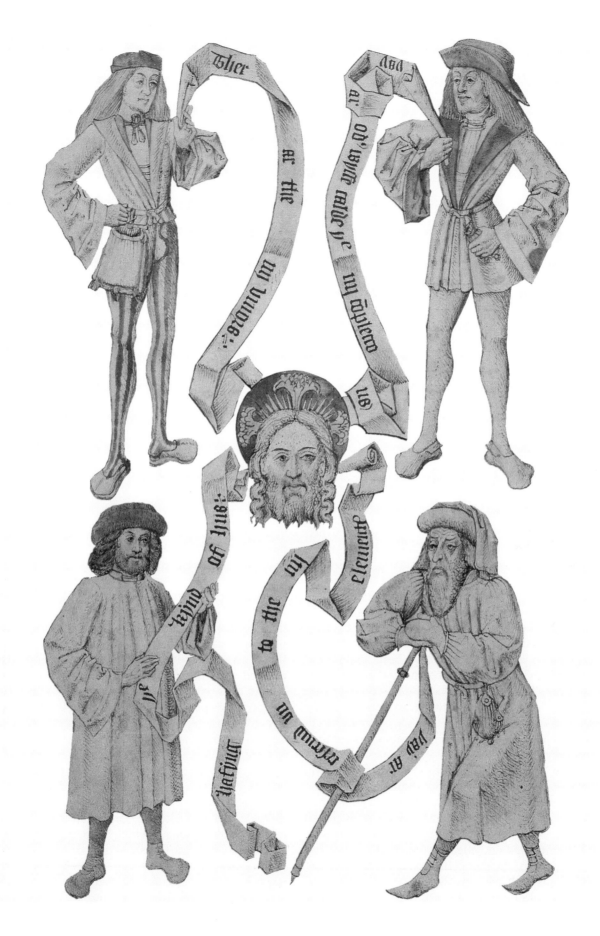

13

Although abhorrent to modern Westerners, cannibalism is in some respects analogous to hormone replacement. Eating parts of the body is a crude reflection of the therapeutic administration of hormones.

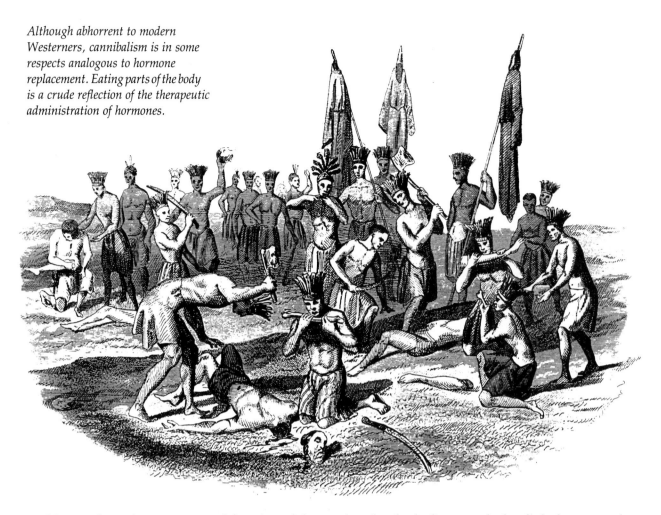

and his work on the anatomy and function of the brain has led to his being called the "first inventor of the nervous system." The system of arteries at the base of the brain is today known as the circle of Willis. Willis is also credited with being the first in modern times to diagnose diabetes by testing the urine for the presence of sugar (although the Chinese used a similar procedure at around A.D. 700). Willis concluded that the best treatment, which at the time was the most medical knowledge could possibly have provided, was undernourishment and lime water. In this way, terminally ill diabetics were given an extra three to six months of life, and it remained a standard treatment until the discovery of insulin.

In 1672 the Swiss scientist Johann Conrad Brunner made an even more remarkable contribution in the field of diabetes when he removed the spleen and pancreas of dogs which he subsequently kept alive, noting thereafter the onset of extreme thirst and sugar in the urine. He had in fact carried out the pioneering experiment that was later to reveal that insulin is secreted by the pancreas, although he did not realize at the time that he had discovered the link between the pancreas and diabetes.

In the eighteenth century, many people had a great impact on the development of endocrinology; Théophile de Bordeu was one of the most important. A Frenchman with a particular interest in the beneficial effects of spas, de Bordeu was years ahead of his time in writing about "emanations" given off by organs throughout the body that entered the blood and brought about distant effects. His view embraced more than just the endocrine glands and is very much in line with the present-day acceptance of hormone secretions from the kidneys, gut and brain.

Another medical giant of the eighteenth century, whose work triggered others to finally unravel much of the mystery of the endocrine system, was the Englishman John Hunter, who was also a brilliant surgeon. Hunter performed a fascinating series of experiments in which he castrated roosters and then observed the shrinking of their combs. Hunter also successfully transplanted birds' testicles, but failed to conclude that the testes were actually releasing secretions into the blood that maintained the secondary sexual characteristics.

More than fifty years passed before another brilliant scientist came to understand and follow up on Hunter's experiments. That scientist was Arnold Berthold, a physician and professor working in Göttingen, Germany. In 1849 he castrated roosters and in some of the birds returned a single testis to the body cavity. Remarkably, he found that the animals carrying a testicular graft exhibited normal sexual behavior and sexual accessories such as the rooster's comb; those that did not receive a graft had withered combs. What really made Berthold's mark in the history of endocrinology, however, was that he concluded from his experiments that the testes released something into the blood which helped maintain male behavior and the secondary sex characteristics.

Mysteriously, Berthold did not follow up his results. It has been suggested that he may have lost interest, or did not appreciate that he had stumbled onto a new field of science. It was in any case another six years before others began to tread the path toward modern endocrinology which Berthold had mapped out. The year 1855 was a watershed in the history of endocrinology, and is regarded by some as the year endocrinology was born as a modern science. In 1855, no fewer than three brilliant scientists earned their places as heroes in endocrinological history.

Claude Bernard of the Collège de France introduced the concept of the ductless gland after showing by chemical methods that the liver could release sugar directly into the blood. He described the process as *sécrétion interne* (internal secretion), as opposed to *sécrétion externe*, meaning the discharge of bile. The Frenchman had stumbled across the key to what was later revealed to be a massive endocrine network.

In the same year Thomas Addison of Guy's Hospital, London, drew attention to a disease of the adrenal glands (now called Addison's disease). He had shrewdly noted the symptoms of poor appetite, low blood pressure, extreme weakness, stomach upsets, and a bronze-colored skin. This was the first endocrine disorder to be accurately diagnosed, and is caused by underactivity of the adrenal glands. Sadly, Addison received little honor in his own country and it was left to the great

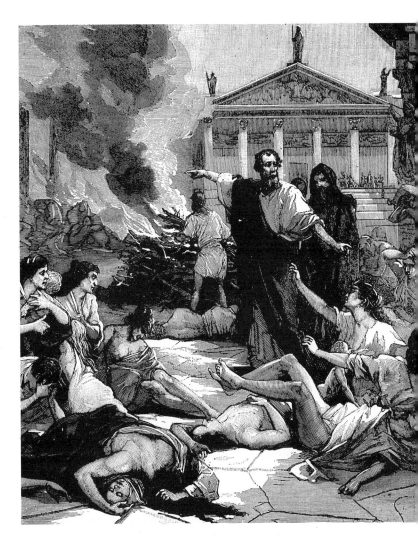

The famous ancient Greek physician Hippocrates — in this old print depicted saving Athenians from a plague — made many notable contributions to medicine. Among these was his notion that the correct balance of the four humors was necessary for good health, a view reflected in the present-day knowledge that the many hormones must each be produced in the correct amounts for proper bodily functioning.

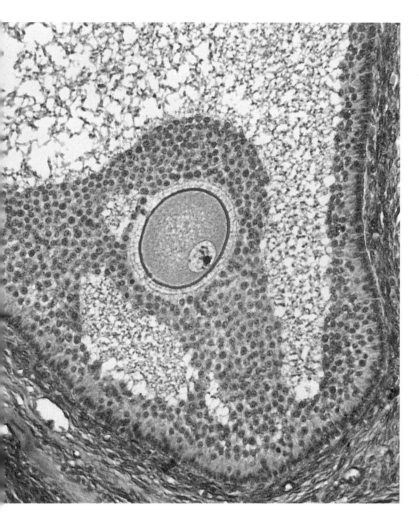

Although we now know that any effect of his "rejuvenation" was most likely due to autosuggestion, his work at the time was greatly admired by others and within two years many physicians were administering testicular extracts.

The year 1889 also saw a significant leap forward in the understanding of diabetes when Joseph von Mering and Oskar Minkowski, two German scientists, observed the onset of diabetes mellitus in a patient after surgical removal of the pancreas.

Sandwiched between the great year of 1885 and the amazing revelations published in 1889 by Brown-Séquard and von Mering and Minkowski, Sir William Gull, a London physician, first established that normal secretion of a gland was essential to good health and that decreased secretion (hyposecretion) led to illness. He was one of the first to classically describe the condition caused by a defective thyroid gland in adulthood (myxedema), a condition which in babies causes stunted growth and impaired mental development.

Gull's discovery was followed by the unraveling of diseases of the pituitary gland by the brilliant French neurologist Pierre Marie, who found that the pituitary gland could become as large as an apple in a patient who presented a particular set of symptoms which he termed *acromégalie*.

In 1891, George Murray, an English physician inspired by the experiments of Brown-Séquard and also by the new understanding of the disease myxedema thanks to William Gull, injected thyroid extract into hypothyroid patients — with remarkably good effect. Murray's simple deduction was that if myxedema was caused by the lack of a substance in the body, then it was "rational treatment" to make up that deficiency by the injection of an extract from a healthy gland. Murray was thus one of the great pioneers of modern hormone replacement therapy.

In 1895 two English scientists, George Oliver and Edward Sharpey-Schafer, demonstrated the blood-pressure-raising effects in dogs after an injection of an extract of the adrenal gland. The active ingredient was later isolated and called epinephrine (adrenaline). The significance of their series of pioneering experiments began a new era in which scientists thereafter tried to determine physiological responses to drugs based on organ extracts.

clinician of the Hôtel-Dieu in Paris, Armand Trousseau, to call the disorder by the name "Addison's disease." Addison, the son of a grocer, felt strongly insulted and deeply hurt by the lack of recognition of his work, and withdrew from medical practice at the age of 65 in 1860, suffering from depression. Later that same year he committed suicide by throwing himself out of a hotel window in Brighton, on England's south coast.

Charles Brown-Séquard, a French physician of mixed French and American ancestry, was inspired by Thomas Addison's work, and by removing the adrenal glands from animals showed how essential the glands were to life. More remarkably, in 1889, he shocked the scientific world by attempting self-rejuvenation by injecting himself with extracts of animal glands. He claimed an astonishing improvement, and enthusiastically described to the Society of Biology in Paris the "remarkable effects produced on myself by subcutaneous injection of a liquid obtained by the maceration on a mortar of the testicle of a dog or of a guinea pig to which one has added a little water."

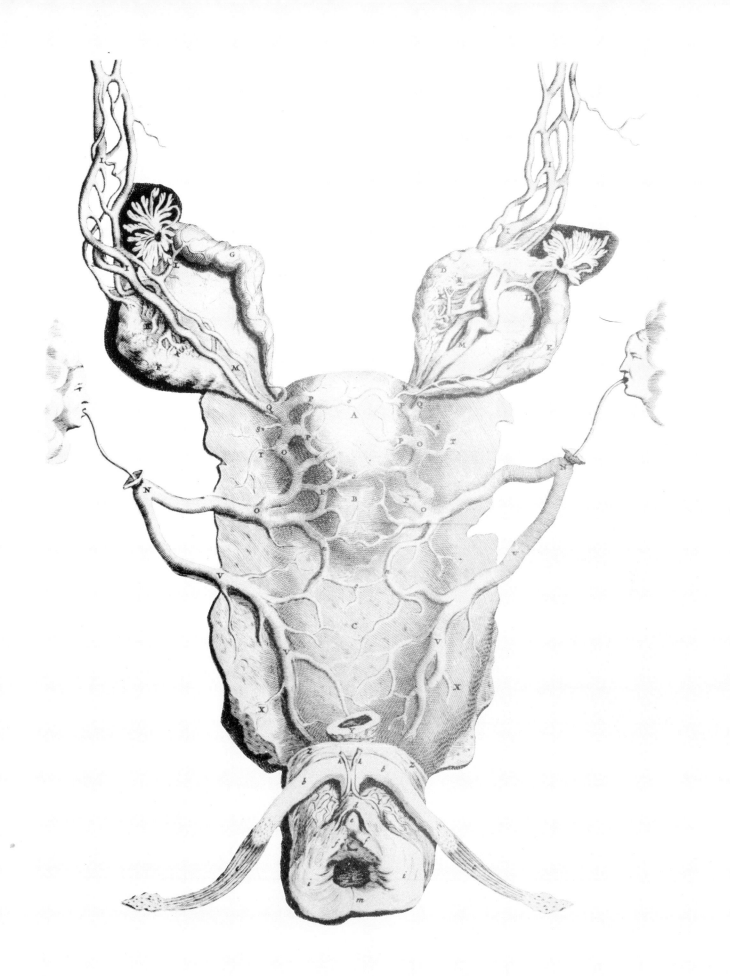

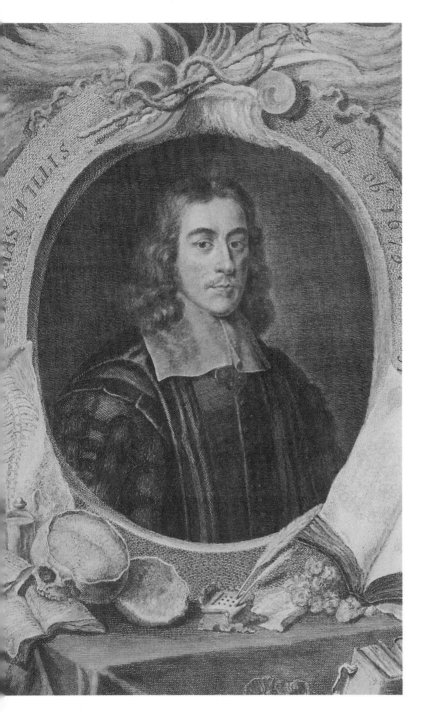

The seventeenth-century English physician Thomas Willis is generally credited with being the first to notice the distinctive sweetness of diabetic urine. This led to his diagnosing diabetes mellitus by testing the urine for the presence of sugar.

Two men in England whose experiments greatly expanded the field of endocrinology were Sir William Bayliss and his friend and colleague Ernest Starling. They managed to show how the hormone secretin was released from the lining of the duodenum in response to the passing of food through the stomach, and then how the hormone, as it passed through the circulation to the pancreas, stimulated the release of pancreatic juices. The concept of chemical messengers was thus born; it was Starling who termed them "hormones" (from the Greek word *hormainō*, meaning "to stir into action"). Starling went on to confirm the suspicions of others that special glands produced chemical messengers to be carried to other organs using the bloodstream as their means of transportation.

The Twentieth Century

The introduction of experimental biochemistry into endocrinology also occurred around the start of the twentieth century. In 1901 Jokichi Takamine and Charles Aldrich, who were working independently of each other in the United States, almost simultaneously succeeded in crystallizing epinephrine. Their pioneering work was the first step along the path toward the isolation and identification of a large number of hormones which today help combat a variety of disorders.

During the next two decades, scientists researching into hormones knew that the pancreas was somehow significant in the disorder of diabetes, and that it secreted a hormone which kept the level of blood sugar normal. What they did not know was that the hormone responsible, insulin, was destroyed by enzymes produced by part of the pancreas during the attempted extraction process. But in Canada Frederick Banting, Charles Best and John MacLeod, and Paulescu in Romania, managed to work around this problem and subsequently were able to isolate highly potent extracts which could reduce the blood sugar levels of experimental animals. The first step in the eventually successful treatment of diabetes was thus made.

For their work, Banting and MacLeod received the Nobel Prize, although Best and Paulescu were not nominated. Bernardo Houssay of Buenos Aires helped to contribute to the understanding of sugar metabolism in the body by demonstrating that

The development and maintenance of roosters' red combs depend on an adequate supply of hormones from the birds' testicles — a discovery made by the German scientist Arnold Berthold in 1849.

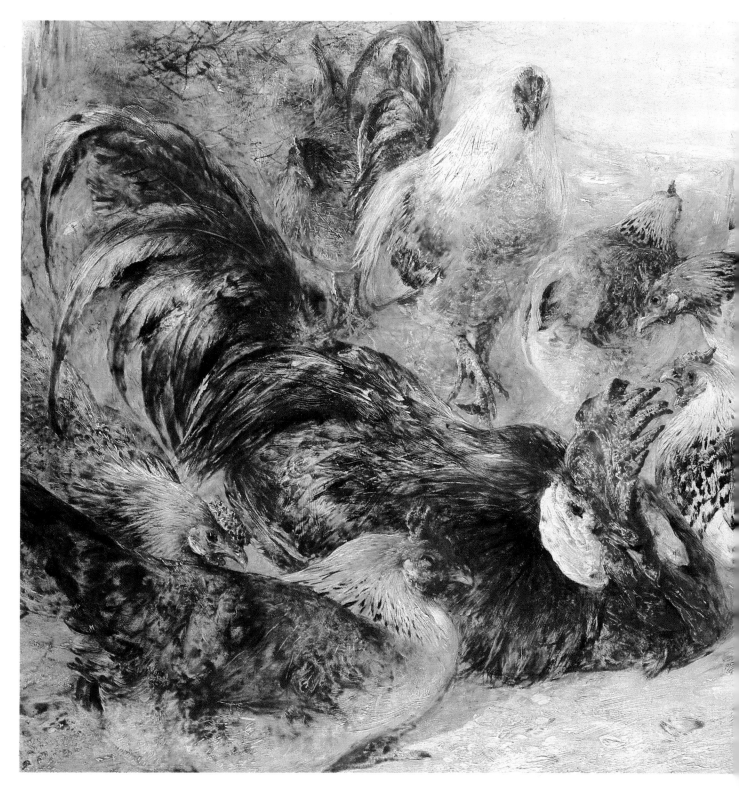

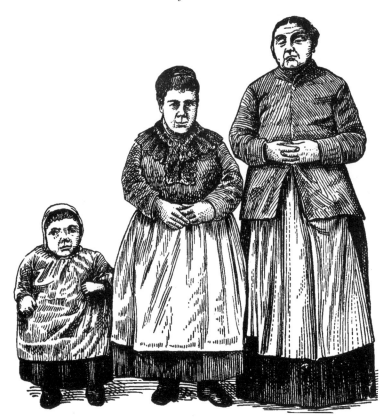

This illustration from Anomalies and Curiosities of Medicine, *published in 1900, shows cases of cretinism and myxedema, the cause of which (thyroid undersecretion) was established 51 years earlier.*

another organ, the anterior pituitary, also had a role to play — a discovery for which he too received a Nobel Prize nearly twenty years later in 1947.

Another gland vital for survival, as established by Brown-Séquard and others, is the adrenal gland. Extracts of the gland could not be administered in large quantities because they contained, in addition to cortisone, the powerful hormone epinephrine, which could be injected safely only in small amounts. Finally, in 1929 it became possible to obtain concentrated extracts of cortisone from the adrenal cortex, without large amounts of epinephrine from the adrenal medulla. As a result, cats from which the adrenal glands had been removed could nevertheless be kept alive with injections of the extracts. This paved the way for the treatment of Addison's disease.

It was not until the mid-1930s, however, that the American biochemist Edward Kendall separated out many of the steroid hormones produced by the adrenal cortex. One of them, named Compound E and later renamed cortisone, has since been used to treat a large number of diseases. Kendall and two of his colleagues were recognized for their magnificent achievement with the award of the Nobel Prize, but it was not until 1949 that Kendall's work really started to make an impact.

It was then that the physician Philip Hench joined forces with Kendall and cautiously announced to the world that cortisone alleviated the symptoms of rheumatoid arthritis. It had been Hench's observation that jaundice and pregnancy could exacerbate rheumatoid arthritis. He concluded that the condition was not caused by infection, as had been thought, but was more likely to be a metabolic disorder. This led to his and Kendall's pioneering experiments on the use of steroids to treat these diseases. An era of steroid investigation had been triggered in which many natural steroid hormones were isolated and subsequently synthesized, thus making them available to physicians.

A leading endocrinologist of the 1930s — and for a long time afterward — was Fuller Albright of Boston who, although suffering from Parkinson's disease at the time, carried out experiments to show the range of debilitating conditions caused by defective parathyroid glands (which are located at the back of the thyroid). It was not until the late 1950s, however, that parathyroid hormone, a vital chemical messenger involved in calcium and phosphorus metabolism, was isolated. In 1962 Douglas Copp discovered a hormone (calcitonin) from the thyroid gland which appeared to act in direct contrast to the parathyroid hormone, thus achieving a regulated effect in the body.

Modern Advances

One of the major events of the 1960s was the development of the radioimmunoassay technique by Rosalyn Yalow and Solomon Berson. This sensitive method of quantification transformed endocrinology, enabling scientists to detect the presence of minute amounts of hormones in the blood. This new technology has aided therapy by enabling physicians to determine the presence of an excess or deficiency of a hormone.

Many new hormones were isolated in the 1960s, and their functions were the subject of feverish activity by scientists who wanted to know not only

Thomas Addison

Early Endocrinologist

It was Thomas Addison's fate for much of his life to be overshadowed by those he worked closely with. Prepared to study and to work hard, even to the extent of joining Guy's Hospital in London as a medical student although he had previously qualified as a physician at Edinburgh University, Addison was the first person to diagnose a certain set of symptoms as the result of changes in the composition or the secretions of an endocrine gland. Essentially, however, he was a loner; an eloquent teacher, his style was somewhat aloof, his disposition subject to bouts of intense introspection, especially later in life.

He was born in Longbenton, to the northeast of Newcastle-upon-Tyne, England, in April 1793. After graduating from Edinburgh in 1815, he moved south to London where he became a surgeon at the Lock Hospital, studying dermatology under Thomas Bateman. It was in 1820 that he entered Guy's Hospital, and he remained there in various senior posts for the rest of his working life.

One of the leading physicians at Guy's was Richard Bright, then celebrated for a number of medical discoveries (including

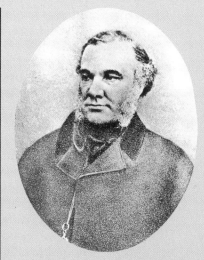

especially the kidney disorder now known as Bright's disease). With Bright and several other scientists at Guy's Addison collaborated both in work and in producing important papers and books.

But it was not until 1849, a full twelve years after Addison had attained the status of physician at Guy's that his diagnosis of the cause of what is now referred to as Addison's disease took place—a discovery from which one commentator has suggested the science of endocrinology itself could be said to date. The medical profession was first informed of it in a lecture to the South London Medical Society. Perhaps because of Addison's own rather haughty style of delivery the lecture was not particularly well received,

and almost instantly forgotten. Called "On anemia: Disease of the suprarenal capsules," the paper related disease of the adrenal glands (the "suprarenal capsules") to the disorder of anemia, as found together in a few autopsies Addison had performed.

Six years later, Addison was still trying to stimulate interest in his discovery, and issued a small book on the subject. By now he was able to include considerably more information, and clearly identified and distinguished the two disorders pernicious anemia (or Addison's anemia) and Addison's disease (of which progressive anemia is one symptom, along with a characteristic bronze coloration of the skin). He was now also able to state that the actual cause of Addison's disease was atrophy of the adrenal cortex (although he did not use such modern terms).

Addison had other claims to the fame that eluded him. With John Morgan he wrote the first handbook on toxicology, and by himself he discovered much of what is now basic knowledge of lobar pneumonia and appendicitis. Yet he was not famous during his life, and finally killed himself, in Brighton, southern England, in June 1860.

Ernest Starling (below) *developed the concept of hormones as chemical messengers as a result of his studies of digestion. In 1902, working with Sir William Bayliss, he discovered that the passage of food through the* *stomach stimulates the release of the hormone secretin from the duodenum* (bottom, *magnified about 70 times), and that this hormone then causes the release of pancreatic fluids. He also coined the term "hormone."* *The praying hands in Albrecht Dürer's drawing show the slight inflammation of the joints that indicates early rheumatoid arthritis. This inflammation may be caused by the action of prostaglandin hormones.*

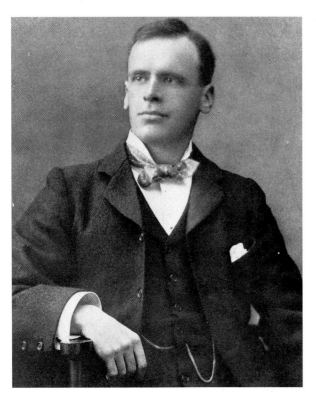

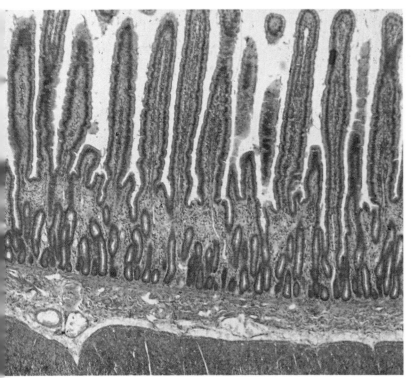

what these substances could do to prevent disease but also how they exerted control over complex processes such as pregnancy. Much of the research into pregnancy went toward developing contraceptive pills — tablets containing hormones such as estrogen and progesterone which effectively alter a woman's menstrual cycle, suppressing ovulation, and thus preventing fertilization of an egg.

During the 1970s and 1980s there have been major advances in contraception using hormones, administered either by injection or by tablet. As scientists learned more about the full process of reproduction it became possible to produce lower-dose contraceptive pills, which are thought to be safer in relation to long-term health.

Another area that has attracted immense attention in recent times is the function of the prostaglandins in the body. Described as probably the most potent and diverse hormones ever to be discovered, they have been found to be significant in many different processes: nervous system function, blood flow in the kidneys, pregnancy, and in the inflammation which occurs in arthritis, to name just a few influences. The endorphins and enkephalins, two groups of hormones found in the brain, are also causing much excitement, even though their precise functions have not yet been fully discerned. They are believed to play an important part in human behavior, however, and may influence the perception of pain.

The study of the ductless glands that produce hormones — the field of endocrinology — has become a specialist subject in its own right. It is known today that the endocrine system is a far more complex and vital system than was thought a century ago. Berthold could not have realized that his idea of internal secretion would lead to such a booming medical field. Even in the early 1960s, the specialty of endocrinology was only just beginning to take a respected foothold in the medical world.

Today endocrinology is still a subject which means different things to different people. Some would regard it as a subject dealing broadly with the chemical integration within living beings, and would include the "local" hormones which do not originate from glands but have local effects near their site of release. Others prefer to follow the classical definition of Bayliss and Starling, who

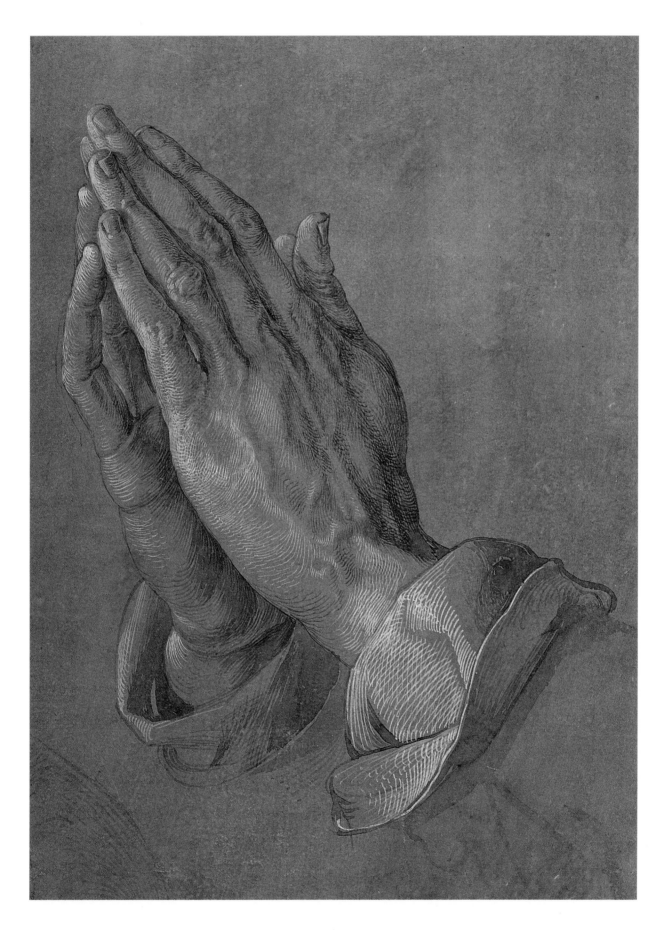

considered the field to include only the secretions and actions of hormones from ductless glands.

Even the term "hormone" has been used more broadly than its classical definition — as proposed by Starling — as a substance released from one part of the body that has a distant effect. But some scientists called the chemicals emanating from wounded tissues "wound hormones," and growth substances in plants which can induce plant growth in areas remote from their site of formation have been called "phytohormones." The latter include auxins, flowering hormones, B vitamins and steroids.

In addition, the nervous system has been shown to be linked to the endocrine system. Nerves can stimulate tissues to release hormones, and chemicals such as acetylcholine (which is released at the end of nerve terminals to allow messages to pass along a nerve network) have been described as neurohormones. The interlocking of the two systems can be considered to constitute a neuroendocrine system.

Without hormones, the chemical messengers which circulate around the body giving instructions to virtually every tissue, we could not live. The endocrine glands pump them into the bloodstream at a rate which they control by marvelous feedback pathways which tell them how the systems they are controlling are performing. Their immense importance to the body in maintaining a stable internal environment includes the regulation of growth, maturation, reproduction, metabolism, and even how the body responds to an emergency. That these hormonal systems are very similar to those of other mammals makes them easy to study, and many of the great endocrinological discoveries have more recently in consequence been made on animals such as dogs and cats.

Endocrine Disorders

As the mysteries of the endocrine system were explained it became apparent that some forms of abnormal physical development, some personality idiosyncrasies, and some mental disorders were linked to variations in endocrine gland activity.

A disorder in a single endocrine gland can have immense consequences for the whole body, often with distressing results. For example, gigantism can be the result of excessive secretion of the growth hormone (somatotropin) by the pituitary gland. Conversely, when the pituitary gland fails to produce enough growth hormone, a midget (a normal dwarf, that is, a dwarf with normal bodily proportions, intelligence and sexual development) is the result.

Not all types of dwarfism result from pituitary deficiency; some have other causes, such as thyroid gland deficiency (hypothyroidism). If hypothyroidism is diagnosed early enough, treatment with thyroid hormone can virtually normalize the child both physically and mentally — but the treatment must be for life. Thyroid deficiency can also occur in adults if the thyroid gland malfunctions. If, on the other hand, the thyroid gland starts to produce an excess of thyroid hormone, the probable result is thyrotoxicosis, accompanied by, nervousness, tremor, sleeplessness and, sometimes, protruding eyes (an effect known as exophthalmic goiter).

Another distressing but related disorder occurs when a person's sex is not clearly defined. Normally, men and women have particular sex hormones specific to their gender responsible for functions such as menstruation, changes during pregnancy, and other reproductive functions. If in the male the sex glands fail to develop normally, a lack of the hormone testosterone leads to poorly developed sex organs and infertility. Conversely, if the sex glands produce an excess of male hormones (in the case of a tumor, for example), puberty is too rapidly advanced for the child's age. Women also naturally produce small amounts of male sex hormones. If the adrenal cortex and ovaries produce too much, a bearded woman is the result; such a woman is also usually well-developed muscularly, and may have a deep and even husky-sounding voice.

Following the revelation of a link between hormones and many disorders, a new era of hormone replacement therapy has occurred since 1970, particularly in view of our new ability to synthesize artificial hormones and produce them via bacteria using new genetic technology of the 1980s. Great progress has certainly been made since ancient and prehistoric humans ate the organs of other humans in what might now be considered the "foretaste" of endocrinology.

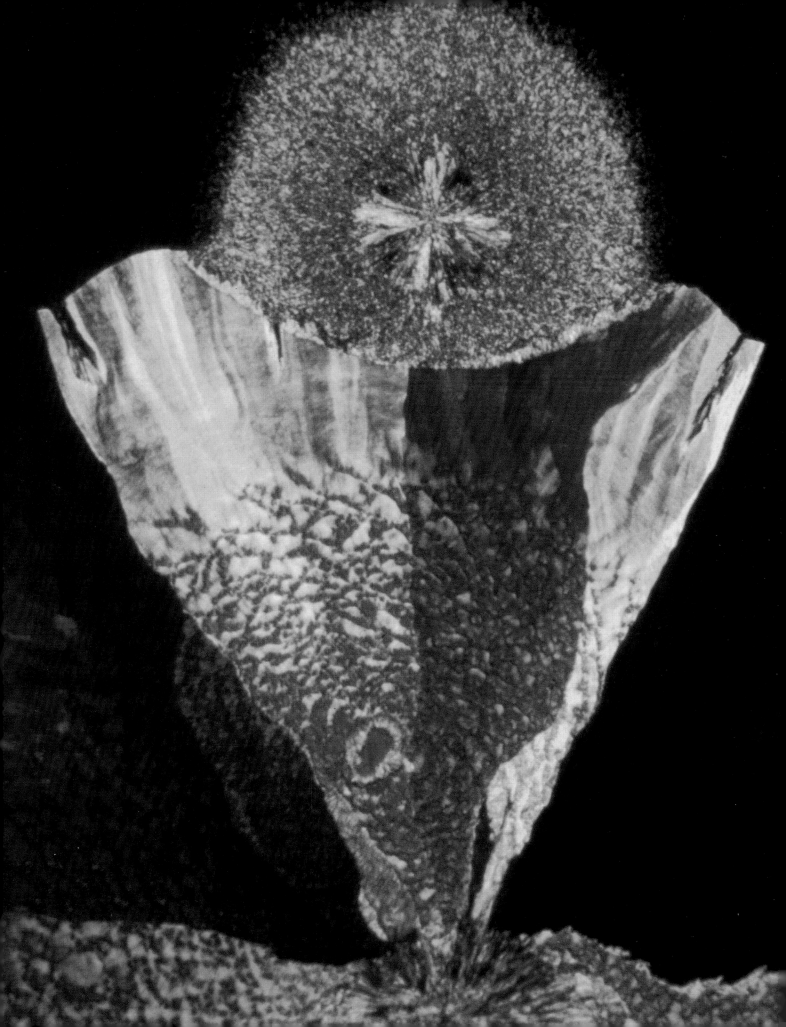

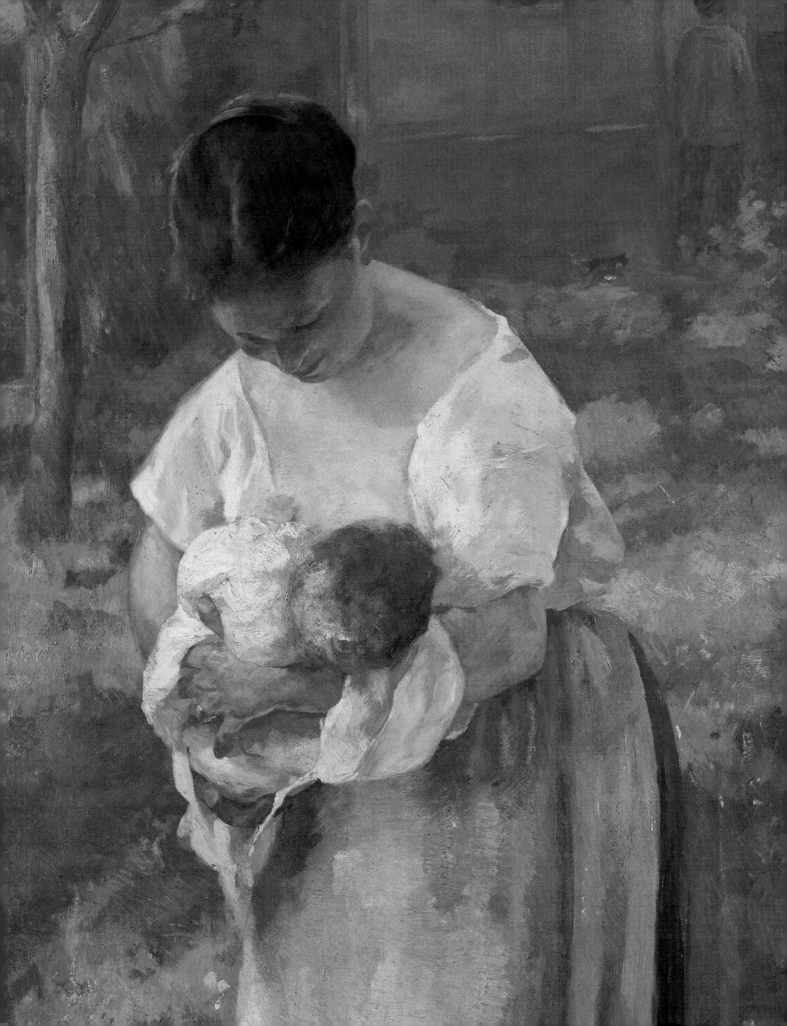

Chapter 2

The Organic Orchestra

In a growing fetus, the endocrine glands develop from the same primitive tissues that give rise to the skin and nervous system. With development, however, the glands become widely separated and are found scattered throughout the body. The endocrine glands are characterized by the fact that they secrete their products directly into the bloodstream or extracellular tissue fluids. Because hormones, the products of endocrine glands, travel via the blood (or tissue fluids) they are able to exert their effects at widespread sites, often at some distance from their source of origin. Some endocrine glands, such as the pancreas, have both endocrine and exocrine functions (some of their secretions are carried in the bloodstream; others travel through ducts) and are therefore referred to as mixed glands.

Although the endocrine glands vary considerably in their gross structures, their microscopic appearances share a number of features. For example, they all have rich blood supplies — a necessity if hormones are to be carried away from them. In addition the blood vessels are specially adapted so that the cells lining them can have hormone-filled granules that open up into the blood capillaries.

The Pituitary Gland

One of the smallest endocrine organs, the pituitary weighs about one-fiftieth of an ounce in an adult and is roughly the size of a pea. It is suspended from the brain by a slender stalk and sits in a bony pocket located just above the back of the nose.

Despite its small size the gland consists of two parts: the anterior pituitary and posterior pituitary. The anterior pituitary produces and secretes no fewer than six different hormones, whereas the posterior produces none of its own. Instead, it consists of nerve cells traveling from the hypothalamus in the brain, carrying two hormones. Thus, although they form part of the same

Breast-feeding a young baby involves two main hormones: prolactin (from the pituitary gland), which stimulates the mother's breast to produce milk, and oxytocin (also from the pituitary), which stimulates the release of milk when the baby sucks on the nipple.

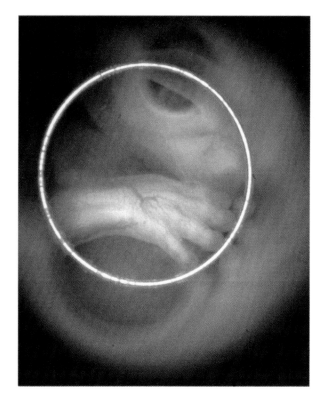

gland, the two lobes of the pituitary have different functions and should therefore be considered separately.

The six hormones secreted by the anterior pituitary gland are prolactin, growth hormone (or somatotropin), corticotropin (or adrenocorticotropin, ACTH), follicle-stimulating hormone (FSH), luteinizing hormone (LH), and thyrotropin (or thyroid-stimulating hormone, TSH). The first two hormones have direct actions of their own, whereas the rest control the activity of other endocrine glands elsewhere in the body. The normal function of prolactin is to stimulate a mother's breast to produce milk and is therefore produced mainly during lactation. Prolactin also interferes with the production or action of the female sex hormones, and this explains why women who are breast-feeding are less likely to have regular menstrual cycles or become pregnant.

In some cases a pituitary tumor may cause the secretion of excess prolactin. In women this results in infertility and the production of milk when it is not required. In fact, in women being investigated for infertility an important test is the measurement of prolactin levels in the blood. The effects of a prolactin-secreting tumor in the male include impotence and loss of sex drive. Most pituitary tumors are small; some cases require surgery, although many may be treated with drugs.

Growth hormone (somatotropin), has an effect on almost every tissue in the body, especially bone and muscle, and is one of the major growth-stimulating hormones. In certain disorders, there may be either excess or insufficient secretion of growth hormone. Frequently, it acts through somatomedin, a hormone synthesized in the liver. Increased production has different effects depending on whether it occurs in children, who have growing bones, or adults. In childhood it results in gigantism; in adults it leads to acromegaly, with characteristic changes to the dimensions of the face, head, hands and feet.

The treatment of these conditions and other pituitary tumors is usually surgery or radiation therapy, although acromegaly may be treated with the drug bromocriptin. Because the pituitary lies very close to the back of the nose, a surgeon is able to operate on it via that route; such an approach was pioneered by the American neurosurgeon Harvey Cushing at the beginning of this century. Powerful new techniques in radiotherapy, including linear accelerators, can in many cases completely avoid the need for an operation. It is not always possible, however, to destroy the tumor without at the same time damaging the rest of the pituitary. For this reason people who have had a tumor treated often need hormone replacement therapy for the rest of their lives.

Not surprisingly, a deficiency of growth hormone has its most serious effect in childhood, when it causes dwarfism. "Pituitary" dwarfs are short, but with normal body proportions, usually sterile, and have normal intelligence. If treated early enough with growth hormone, pituitary dwarfs can attain normal height and fertility.

. The other four hormones secreted by the anterior pituitary exert profound effects on other endocrine glands. Corticotropin stimulates secretion of glucocorticoids such as cortisone by the adrenal cortex, and thyrotropin stimulates the thyroid gland to produce its hormones. Follicle-stimulating

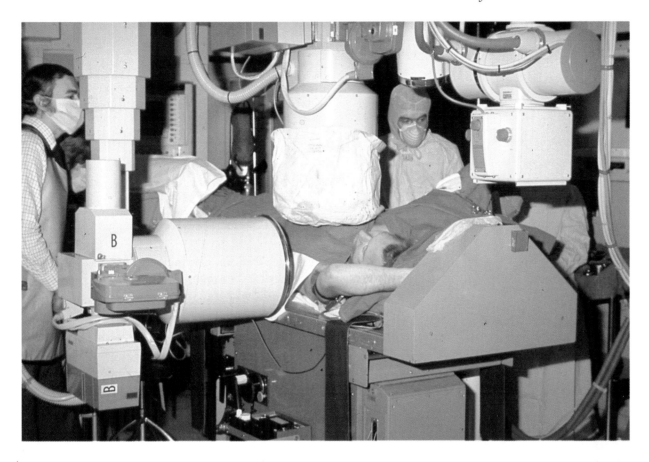

hormone and luteinizing hormone are known as the gonadotropins because they act on the male and female reproductive glands.

Like a thermostat, the pituitary secretion of these four hormones is under feedback control. In the case of corticotropin its production by the pituitary results in the increased secretion of glucocorticoids by the adrenals. In addition to their many biological effects, glucocorticoids act on the pituitary to inhibit the further production of corticotropin. In this way the blood levels of glucocorticoids are kept under control.

Very similar feedback mechanisms regulate the blood levels of the other pituitary hormones. The situation is further complicated by the fact that secretion of these hormones is itself under the control of other hormones originating in the hypothalamus, which reach the pituitary by means of small blood vessels in the stalk that suspends the pituitary from the brain.

The two hormones produced by the hypothalamus and stored in the posterior pituitary — which develops as a downgrowth of brain substance — are oxytocin and vasopressin (or antidiuretic hormone, ADH). Oxytocin stimulates the contraction of smooth muscle, especially of the uterus, and is particularly important at the end of pregnancy. It is one of the factors that cause the uterus to contract at the time of delivery. In fact, one way of inducing labor at the end of a normal pregnancy is to administer oxytocin.

Oxytocin also stimulates contraction of the muscle cells that surround the milk-producing glands of the breast. When a baby sucks on the mother's nipple a reflex action, involving centers in the mother's brain, results in increased oxytocin release. This in turn causes the contraction of the muscle cells of the breast and consequently the release of milk. The additional oxytocin secreted in response to suckling causes further contractions of

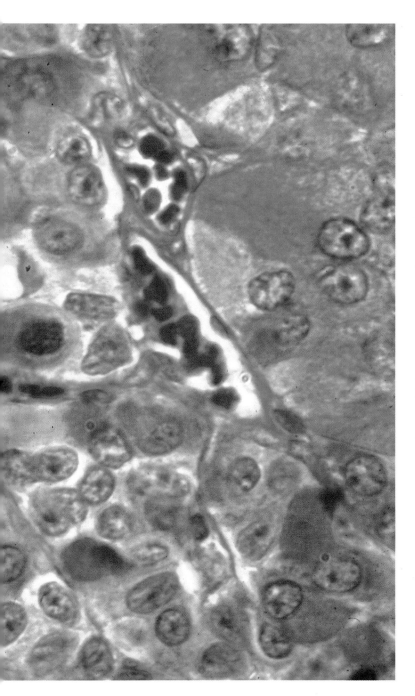

A beautifully counterstained section of part of the pituitary gland reveals its constituent cell types in this photomicrograph. The pituitary is one of the smallest endocrine glands —being about the size of a pea—but secretes six different hormones from its anterior or front part, and stores and releases two other hormones from its posterior or rear portion.

the uterus, and thereby also assists in the ejection of the placenta immediately following birth.

The Pancreas and Islets of Langerhans

One of the body's least accessible organs, the pancreas is located at the back of the abdomen, just underneath the stomach and in front of the vertebral column. It has two distinct components: the bulk of the gland, which secretes enzymes involved in the digestion of food, and an enormous number of small islands of cells, which secrete hormones. The pancreas has approximately two million such islets, which are named for the German anatomist Paul Langerhans, although he did not realize the function of these cells. It was the French physician Étienne Lancereaux who noted a relationship between the pancreas and the disease he called diabetes mellitus.

Diabetes Mellitus

This condition is characterized by increased intake of fluid, together with excretion of excessive quantities of urine which contains glucose, and weight loss.

In 1921 a young orthopedic surgeon named Frederick Banting together with a Professor of Physiology, John MacLeod, and a medical student, Charles Best, started on a series of experiments using dogs with the aim of identifying which component of the pancreas was involved in the control of blood sugar (already named insulin even before it had been isolated). Soon after graduation, Banting was excited by a publication which described an experiment in which the duct of the pancreas, through which its digestive juices drain to the intestine, was tied off. This produced almost complete degeneration of the pancreas except for the islets of Langerhans.

Banting's idea was that previous injections of pancreatic extracts had been unreliable because of the effect of the digestive enzymes on insulin. By using the tied-off pancreases, he and his co-workers were able to obtain almost pure extracts of insulin from the islets of Langerhans. Thanks to Best's biochemical training before becoming a medical student, they were able to isolate insulin in a relatively pure form. They then turned their attention to obtaining insulin from cattle. The

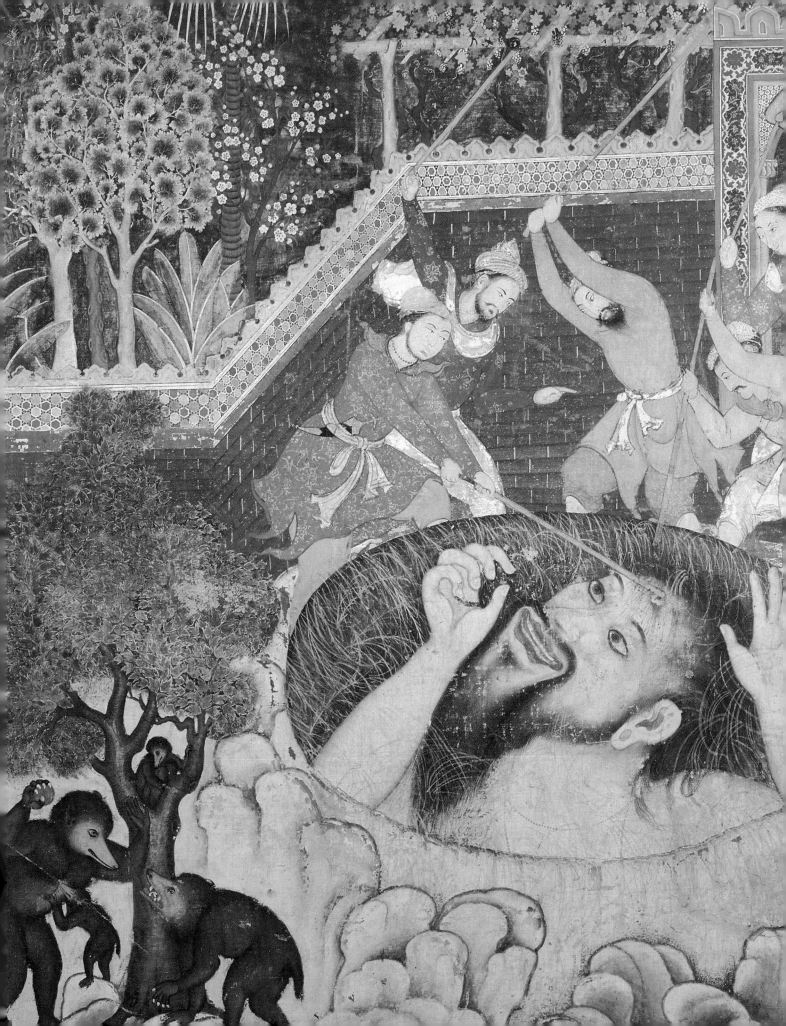

In many cases hormone secretion is regulated by a negative feedback mechanism, whereby one gland produces a hormone that stimulates a second gland to produce another hormone—which has an inhibitory effect on hormone secretion by the first gland. The diagram below illustrates the feedback process that controls corticotropin secretion by the pituitary. Corticotropin stimulates the adrenals to increase their secretion of glucocorticoids which, in addition to affecting the level of sugar in the blood, also inhibit the further production of corticotropin. The effect is to maintain a constant level of corticotropin.

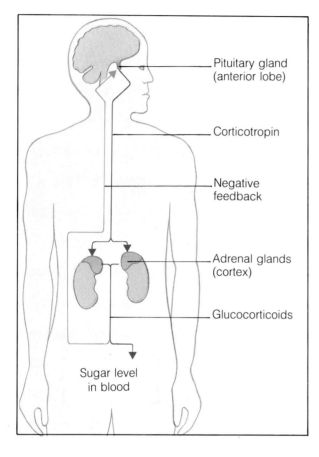

Pituitary gland (anterior lobe)

Corticotropin

Negative feedback

Adrenal glands (cortex)

Glucocorticoids

Sugar level in blood

blood (because it causes the breakdown of fats and proteins) and tends to be secreted at times of stress.

Diabetes is caused either by inadequate secretion of insulin in the pancreas or by resistance of the body to the hormone's action. The first type, due to the failure of insulin production, is more common in children. It tends to appear suddenly and is associated with a severe metabolic upset. The second type, due to unresponsiveness to insulin, usually occurs in older, often overweight, patients and tends to have a milder course.

Diabetes has been described as "starvation in the midst of plenty." This refers to the accumulation of glucose in the blood caused by its failure to enter the tissues, which as a result, are starved of their major energy source. Excess sugar in the blood spills out into the urine, increasing the overall volume produced. Fluid loss and extreme thirst occur as a result.

Diabetics may suffer from a variety of symptoms ranging from coma to more insidious complications. It is the insidious complications that are more difficult to control. They tend to involve all parts of the body, especially the eyes, kidneys, heart and blood vessels. Diabetes may damage the eyes in a number of ways. It may do so by causing the lens to become opaque (a cataract) or by damaging the retina, the light-sensitive layer at the back of the eye. This is one of the most common causes of blindness (defined as a visual acuity of less than 29 per cent) in the United States. Kidney failure is relatively common in young diabetics and, like most of the complications of diabetes, is more common in patients who have suffered from the disease for a long time. Heart attacks occur more frequently and at younger ages in diabetics than in the rest of the population because the disorder is associated with narrowing of the coronary arteries. Other arteries may also be affected and sometimes if an artery to an extremity — a hand or foot — becomes closed off altogether, gangrene may develop, requiring the amputation of that limb.

The life expectancy of diabetics, especially those who have the disease from childhood, has been markedly improved by the availability of insulin. The hormone cannot be taken orally because, being a protein, it would be digested. It is therefore given by injection, usually twice a day into the thigh or

material obtained in this way proved safe and effective when administered to human diabetics. Once rapidly fatal in some patients, diabetes can now be controlled. An illustration of the effectiveness of this treatment is that one of the first patients to receive beef insulin in 1922 lived a full life for sixty further years.

It is now known that in addition to insulin, the pancreatic islets also secrete another hormone called glucagon. The two hormones are secreted by different cell types: insulin by beta cells, and glucagon by alpha cells. Surprisingly, perhaps, the hormones have opposite effects on blood glucose. Insulin lowers the amount of glucose in the blood by facilitating the entry of glucose into the cells of the body. In addition, it is important in the manufacture and storage of fats and proteins and, by stimulating the production of large molecules from small ones, in growth. Glucagon, in contrast, increases the amount of glucose present in the

Hormones play a central role during pregnancy. After the fertilized egg has implanted in the uterine wall, it produces chorionic gonadotropin. This hormone keeps the corpus luteum intact and so enables it to continue secreting progesterone for about the first three months of pregnancy. During this time the placenta develops and produces estrogen, progesterone and gonadotropin. Just before and during labor the amount of oxytocin (from the pituitary) increases, which stimulates contractions of the womb and also the flow of milk into ducts behind the nipples. After delivery, prolactin maintains milk secretion.

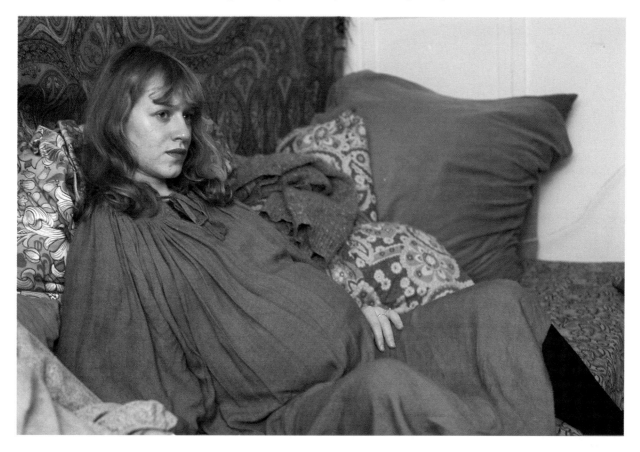

abdomen. Older patients with the lesser form of diabetes respond to drugs termed oral hypoglycemic agents, which increase their responsiveness to their own insulin. Many such people have only a mild form of the disease which can be controlled by diet alone. Overweight patients can often control the disease merely by losing weight — perhaps by abandoning a comfortable life style.

The most common types of insulin used are derived from the pancreas glands of cows or pigs. The human body normally tolerates them well, but a minority of patients have allergic reactions. For these people human-type insulins (products of the rapid modern advances in techniques of genetic engineering) are available.

Diabetes mellitus should be distinguished from another much less common condition also associated with an excessive production of urine —diabetes insipidus. This is caused by failure of the hypothalamus and posterior pituitary to secrete vasopressin (antidiuretic hormone), so that water cannot be reabsorbed by the kidney.

The Thyroid

Controller of the body's metabolism, the thyroid is a fleshy gland located in the neck just below the larynx and in front of the windpipe. It is composed of follicles lined by a single layer of epithelium, surrounding central material called colloid. Colloid contains the carbohydrate–protein complex thyroglobulin, which is converted by the follicular cells into the hormones thyroxine (T_4) and tri-iodothyronine (T_3). The follicle cells are stimulated into activity by thyrotropin, or thyroid-stimulating hormone (TSH), from the anterior pituitary. The hormones are absorbed into capillaries at the base of these cells and then carried by the bloodstream to the rest of the body.

The first step in the synthesis of T_4 and T_3 is the trapping of iodine within the gland. The thyroid

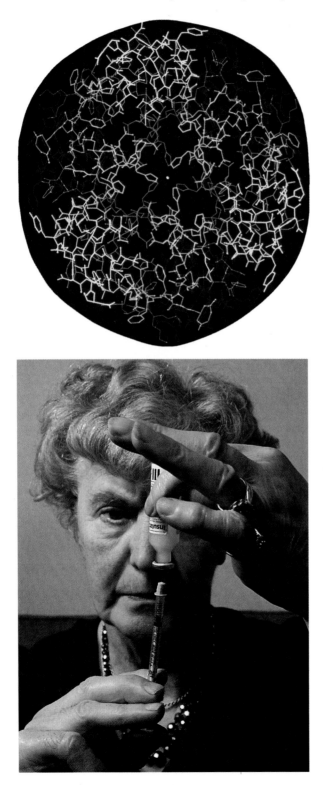

has a remarkable ability to concentrate iodine taken in with the diet. In the thyroid iodine is combined with amino acids to form T_4 and T_3 thyroid hormones. Those in the blood are bound to proteins. The small amounts of free hormones present are able to influence the rates of activity of virtually all the cells in the body; the protein-bound hormone acts as a reserve supply. The hormones also exert negative feedback control on the hypothalamus and the pituitary, which controls the levels of T_3 and T_4 through TSH. T_3 is thought to work at the cellular level, T_4 is converted to T_3 in other parts of the body and acts as an additional thyroid hormone reservoir.

Between the follicular cells of the thyroid lie cells of another type, called parafollicular cells or C cells. Their function remained a mystery until 1962, but they are now known to have an endocrine function and to secrete the hormone calcitonin. It has the effect of lowering the level of calcium in the blood.

Enlargement of the thyroid is much more common in females than in males. Other than diabetes, thyroid disease is the most common endocrine disorder.

One of the first medical descriptions of thyroid hypofunction involving children came from the sixteenth-century Swiss alchemist and physician Paracelsus who described a condition that came to be referred to as cretinism. The corresponding condition in adults is called myxedema.

Excessive activity of the thyroid gland leads to hyperthyroidism or thyrotoxicosis. The term Graves' disease is used to describe a type of excessive thyroid activity characterized by a generalized enlargement of the gland (leading to a swollen neck) and, often, protruding eyes.

The swelling accompanying enlargement of the thyroid gland is called a goiter. In addition to Graves' disease, causes include enhanced activity of the thyroid at times of increased metabolic requirements, especially during puberty and pregnancy. The thyroid gland enlarges because of stimulation by increased levels of TSH in an attempt to increase the thyroid's efficiency at trapping iodine and maintaining normal levels of thyroid hormones. If iodine deficiency exists and is severe, the thyroid is unable to compensate and hypothyroidism results.

Banting, Best and MacLeod

Isolating Insulin

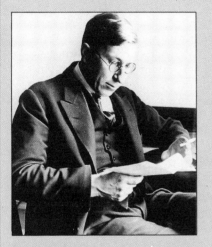 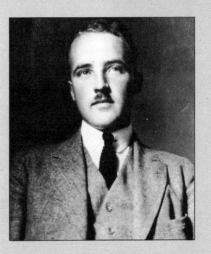 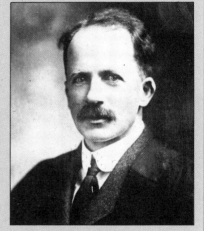

Frederick Grant Banting was undoubtedly the inspiration behind the isolation of insulin for use in the treatment of diabetes. He and John James Rickard MacLeod shared the Nobel Prize in medicine for its discovery.

Banting was a war hero, a medical officer awarded the Military Cross for gallantry during World War I. Returning to his native Canada he took up medical practice, and in 1921—at the age of 30—he started research into diabetes at the University of Toronto. At that time the disease was almost always fatal. A hormone—the lack of which caused all the diabetic symptoms— was known to be secreted somehow by the pancreas and, because it was suspected of being formed by the islets of Langerhans, had

already been named insulin (from the Latin for island), although it had not then been isolated.

Banting had an idea, and with it approached the head of the Physiology Department at the University, John MacLeod, already an authoritative figure renowned for studies of carbohydrate metabolism. MacLeod helped Banting by making available some dogs on which to perform experiments, the laboratory space to carry them out, and an assistant— Charles Herbert Best, a graduate student some eight years younger than Banting.

Banting's notion was to tie the pancreatic ducts of one group of dogs (causing degeneration of pancreas tissue, except for the islets of Langerhans, and so possibly isolating insulin), and to

remove the pancreases entirely from a second group (causing a diabetes-type condition). The diabetic dogs were then injected with a saline extract from the pancreases of the first group. The idea was proved right: their condition improved.

The next step was to obtain a purer form for human use. A young chemist called V. B. Collip helped considerably in this. Success was announced early in 1922, and insulin thereafter revolutionized the treatment of diabetes.

Banting insisted on sharing his part of the Nobel Prize with Best, and crediting Collip. He was knighted in 1934, after the foundation of the Banting-Best Department of Medicine Research at Toronto University, which Best went on to direct after Banting's death in an airplane crash in 1941.

In regions where there is a deficiency of iodine in the soil — and therefore in the diets of local people — goiters are particularly frequent. For this reason, it is common in mountainous parts of the world such as the Andes and the Himalayas (although it has been eliminated completely from other areas such as Salt Lake City, Utah, by the addition of iodine compounds to the common table salt people buy in shops).

To try to detect cases of hypothyroidism at a time when treatment can be of maximum benefit, a baby's TSH levels are usually measured soon after birth. In the first month of life the condition is associated with sleepiness and feeding problems. In the following months physical and mental impairment become apparent; deafness is especially common. Treatment should be begun early with the administration of thyroxine, following which dramatic improvements can be observed.

Myxedema, deficiency of thyroid hormones in an adult, can have various causes, ranging from iodine deficiency to destruction of part of the thyroid by surgery, radiation therapy or inflammation. The development of hypothyroidism following treatment of thyrotoxicosis is a frequent cause of this condition.

Hashimoto's disease was first described by the Japanese surgeon Hakaru Hashimoto. It usually affects middle-aged women, who develop a goiter from infiltration of the thyroid gland by enormous numbers of white blood cells called lymphocytes. The relationship between this type of white cell and damage to the thyroid gland resulting in hypothyroidism has been made clearer by researchers working at the Middlesex Hospital in London. They showed that the white cells produce antibodies which cause the damage — an example of an autoimmune disease. Such self-directed immunity disorders can also affect other endocrine organs and tend to occur together. In some people there is a genetic predisposition to them, or they may be precipitated by a viral infection.

The symptoms of myxedema include a hoarse voice, tiredness, weight gain, cold intolerance, depression, dry skin and loss of hair, infertility, heavy or extended menstruation in women, and constipation. The mental disturbances rarely predominate and if severe are sometimes referred

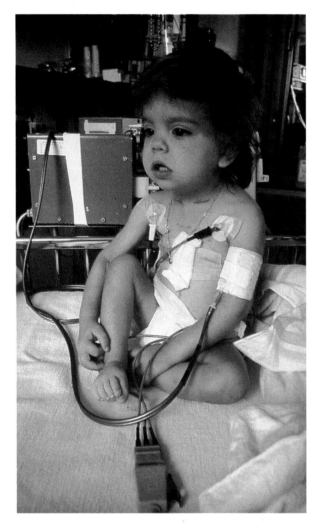

Diabetes mellitus may cause various complications, including kidney failure, which is relatively common in young diabetics. In some cases the kidneys may fail completely, as with this young girl, who is undergoing dialysis to rid her blood of the toxic substances the kidneys normally remove.

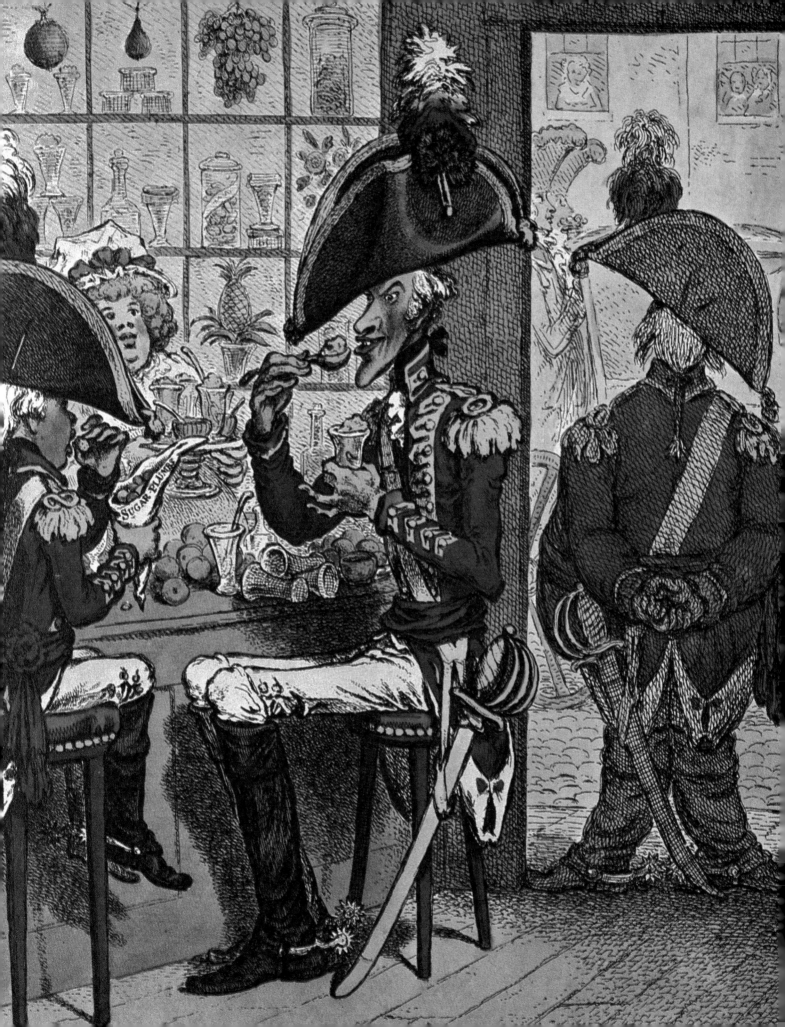

The lens of the eye can become opaque (with a cataract) as a result of diabetes. Fortunately, vision can usually be restored by removal of the lens, although the patient needs eyeglasses thereafter.

The specialized technique of fluorescence microscopy gives this unusual view of thyroid tissue. The thyroid packages and stores large amounts of its hormones in a inactive form.

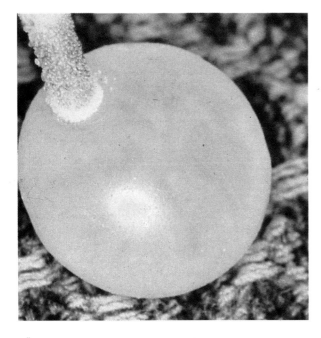

to as "myxedema madness." The accumulation of mucous material within the skin leads to coarsening of the features. One curious feature is that elderly patients with hypothyroidism often do not show whitening of their hair.

Myxedema is diagnosed by measuring blood levels of TSH (which are usually high) and thyroxine and triiodothyronine (which are always low). In cases of thyroid malfunction caused by pituitary or hypothalamic failure there are decreased levels of TSH. Treatment involves the oral administration of thyroxine, which of course must be continued for life.

Hyperthyroidism or thyrotoxicosis has several causes. The form known as Graves' disease most frequently occurs in young women, and may be due to an autoimmune process in which an antibody stimulates the thyroid cells. The characteristic staring appearance is caused by retraction of the eyelids, sometimes accompanied by inflammation of the ocular muscles, which in turn causes protrusion of the eyes. Recent research suggests that Graves' disease may in some cases transform into Hashimoto's disease.

The result of increased circulating levels of thyroxine and triiodothyronine is that almost all the tissues in the body are stimulated to become hyperactive. An increase in metabolic rate causes weight loss (despite a good appetite) and excessive sweating together with an inability to tolerate heat. Cardiac problems are common, and palpitations and fast heart rate may occur. Patients may become emotionally upset and in some cases display a type of psychosis.

Treatment of thyrotoxicosis is often with drugs such as methimazole or propylthiouracil that block the synthesis of the thyroid hormones. Drug therapy may be continued for up to one or two years, or a few months may be sufficient. Surgery is preferred in some adult cases. If the thyroid is markedly enlarged, special care must be taken because during the operation large amounts of thyroid hormones may be released into the circulation, leading to a "thyroid crisis;" to avoid such a catastrophic event antithyroid drugs and iodine are normally administered to patients before the operation.

Besides surgery and drugs, another method of treating thyrotoxicosis in a non-pregnant adult is to administer radioactive iodine. This is preferentially taken up by the overactive thyroid, and part of the gland is destroyed. With either surgery or radioactive iodine, a common result is an underactive thyroid. The patient then requires replacement therapy with thyroid hormone.

Thyroiditis, inflammation of the thyroid gland, is not uncommon, and may be caused by viral infections such as mumps. Cancer of the thyroid is fairly frequent, and is often an incidental finding in patients being treated for other disorders. Thyroid tumors are generally slow-growing, and readily treated by surgery, administration of radioactive iodine, or suppression of tumor growth with thyroid hormone. With currently available treatments the life expectancy is good for all patients except those with the most aggressive types of cancer.

Experiments on calcium metabolism in dogs first led to the identification of calcitonin as an agent important in controlling calcium levels in the body. Initially it was thought to be produced not by the thyroid gland but by the closely related parathyroids. Only in the early 1960s was it shown in fact to come from the thyroid. It was also shown that calcitonin is produced by the parafollicular

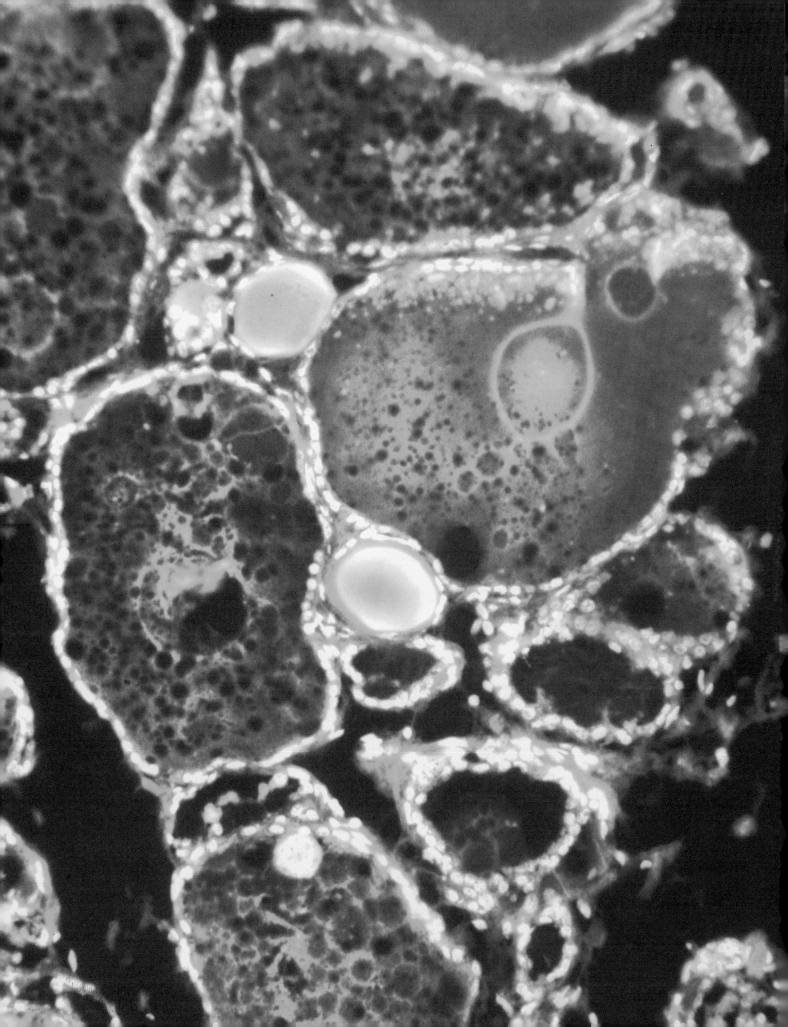

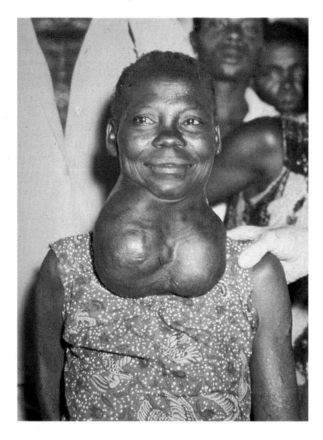

central role for the parathyroids in the metabolism of these two substances, both of which are necessary for maintaining the normal structure and continued health of bones.

The first person to describe the disease caused by overactivity of the parathyroid gland was Friedrich von Recklinghausen. In 1891, while Professor of Pathology at Strasbourg, he described a generalized softening of the bones associated with cyst formation and the laying down of fibrous tissue in the bone marrow, a condition known as von Recklinghausen's disease of bone. Overactivity of the parathyroids is usually caused by an adenoma (a benign tumor), which is generally treated by surgery. The condition is usually detected by the finding of an elevated level of blood calcium in someone who displays no other symptoms and has a blood analysis for an unconnected reason.

Like other endocrine disorders, malfunction of the parathyroid glands may take the form of decreased activity (hypoparathyroidism) or over-activity (hyperparathyroidism). One of the causes of hypoparathyroidism is damage to or removal of the glands, which may occur during surgery on the nearby thyroid gland. It is therefore necessary to monitor patients' blood calcium carefully in the days or weeks after surgery to prevent the development of complications such as muscle cramps or, in severe cases, tetany, which may include spasm of the larynx leading to the danger of asphyxia after surgery on the neck.

Hypoparathyroidism is not treated by administering parathormone, the hormone produced by this gland, which is difficult to purify and thus expensive, but by giving calcium and vitamin D. The calcium may be administered in the form of tablets or by increasing the dietary intake of dairy products, which are rich in calcium.

Increased levels of parathyroid hormone result in mobilization of calcium from its major store in the bones and increases the excretion of phosphate by the kidney. It increases the activity of vitamin D, which is also important in the metabolism of calcium and bone. The results of the raised serum calcium causes symptoms characterized by "stones, bones and groans": kidney stones, bone disease, and pain from both. Kidney stones are a frequent feature of hyperparathyroidism, and

cells. Calcitonin is relatively infrequently associated with clinical problems. Even tumors causing its overproduction are not associated with serious abnormalities in calcium metabolism.

Parathyroid Glands

There are four parathyroid glands, taking the form of brownish pea-sized structures attached to the back of the thyroid gland. They were first identified in 1850 by the English anatomist Sir Richard Owen, who found them in a rhinoceros which had died in a zoo. Thirty years later they were located in humans. The removal of the parathyroids from animals results in tetany, a condition in which muscles in different parts of the body go into continued spasms. The condition occurs also in humans, generally in association with low levels of calcium in the blood, but it may have other causes. Removal of the parathyroids is associated with a decrease in the level of calcium in the blood and a simultaneous rise in phosphorus. This indicates a

40

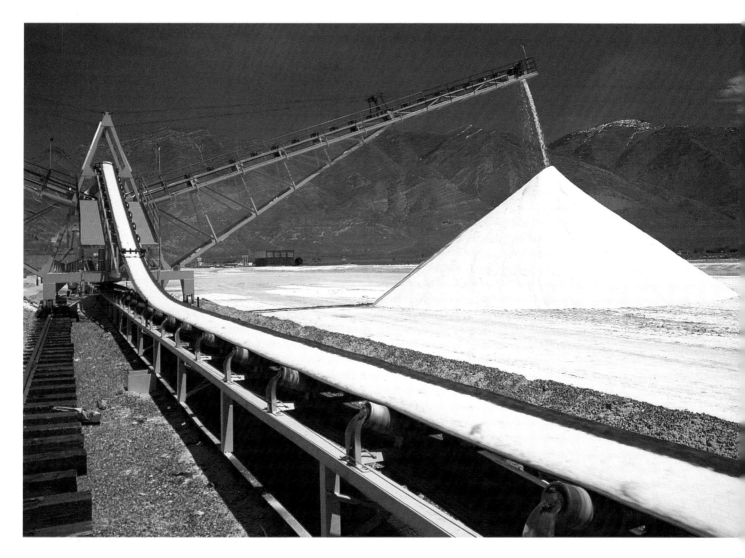

patients with stones need to have their blood calcium levels measured.

Adrenal Glands

The adrenals are two small glands, roughly triangular in shape, which are located on the upper part of each kidney; this accounts for their alternative name of suprarenal glands. Each adrenal consists of two relatively discrete parts: an outer yellow cortex and an inner orange-brown medulla. The cortex is itself made up of three zones, and in a fetus a fourth one is situated between the other three and the medulla. This additional zone disappears soon after birth and its function is unclear. The three adult zones of the adrenal cortex are the outer one, which is responsible for the secretion of mineralocorticoids (steroid hormones that regulate fluid and mineral balance) and the inner two that produce glucocorticoids (which are not only important in controlling the metabolism of glucose but have a wide variety of other functions).

The adrenal cortex also secretes, even in females, male sex hormones (androgens).

The centrally located adrenal medulla, unlike the cortex, is derived from neural tissue and secretes epinephrine and norepinephrine. The hormones secreted by the medulla exert widespread effects on vascular tone, on the heart, and on the nervous system, as well as also affecting glucose metabolism. Together the adrenal cortex and medulla are central to the body's response to stress.

The adrenal glands were first identified during the Middle Ages but approximately 300 more years had to pass before Thomas Addison — who is considered by many to be the founder of endocrinology — working in Guy's Hospital in London, published a book about diseases of the adrenals in which he distinguished atrophy of the adrenal gland (Addison's disease) from pernicious anemia. During the late 1930s the American Edward Kendall and the Swiss Tadens Reichstein working at the Mayo Clinic identified most of the substances produced by the cortex, the steroids or glucocorticoids, which have complex structures. One such steroid is cortisone.

Adrenal atrophy is caused by damage to the cortex. In the past and today in the Third World, tuberculosis was the commonest cause. The most frequent cause now is an autoimmune process which results from adrenocortical destruction by the body brought about by antibodies and white cells. It often occurs with other autoimmune diseases (evident, for example, with Hashimoto's disease of the thyroid).

The common clinical features of adrenal insufficiency include dark pigmentation of the skin and a variety of nonspecific symptoms such as weakness, weight loss and dizziness. The somber pigmentation is seen especially in the skin of scars and the mouth. It may appear either suddenly, particularly associated with episodes of stress, or over a long period of time. President John F. Kennedy was diagnosed as having Addison's disease, which necessitated the administration of glucocorticoids. A difficulty commonly encountered by physicians ·in balancing a patient's requirements for glucocorticoids — which vary considerably according to the amount of stress such as infection or trauma — is illustrated by his case. Photographs indicate that during his election campaign he developed the symptoms of glucocorticoid excess (Cushing's syndrome) as a result of the failure to achieve the correct dosage in the face of hectic activity.

Investigation for the presence of Addison's disease involves tests to see if the adrenal glands can respond to the injection of ACTH by an increased production of glucocorticoids. (With this disease, the adrenal cortex is typically unable to do so.) An important factor for physicians to consider when measuring the levels of corticosteroids in the blood is that levels tend to be higher in the morning than in the evening. Treatment involves the lifelong intake of hydrocortisone. It is important to increase the intake during episodes of infection and surgery to cope with stress.

Excess secretion of glucocorticoids, Cushing's syndrome, is in many cases caused by excess secretion of ACTH from a pituitary tumor. Increased secretion of corticosteroids may also be caused by a tumor of the adrenal cortex and by increasingly well recognized secretion of ACTH-like substances by tumors, especially of the lung. Patients with Cushing's syndrome are often obese — a condition characterized by a moon face, buffalo hump at the neck and protruberant abdomen with relatively thin legs — and may have stretch marks, a tendency to bleed, high blood pressure, weakness, psychiatric disturbances, impaired reproductive function, back pain and diabetes mellitus.

Glucocorticoids are now administered to treat many diseases, especially a number of disorders characterized by inappropriate inflammation. This is because corticosteroids have a remarkable ability to suppress the inflammatory process seen in conditions ranging from asthma to rheumatoid arthritis. It was for his use of steroids in treating the symptoms of rheumatoid arthritis, that Philip Hench shared Kendall and Reichstein's Nobel Prize in 1950. Unfortunately it was only later realized that the side effects of administering large amounts of glucocorticoids (such as hydrocortisone) are those of Cushing's disease and include such serious problems as growth retardation in children and vertebral collapse in adults. Thus although glucocorticoids do have extremely useful applications, physicians have to be very careful to keep the dosage down to a minimum.

In addition to overproduction of glucocorticoids the adrenal cortex, in certain conditions, secretes excess quantities of one of its other two products, mineralocorticoids or androgens. The overproduction of mineralocorticoids is termed Conn's syndrome and is most commonly caused by a small benign tumor of the adrenal cortex. Excess of mineralocorticoids, especially aldosterone, causes retention of sodium and water, leading to raised blood pressure. Contrary to the American internist Jerome Conn's early claims, Conn's syndrome is a relatively rare reason for high blood pressure.

Excess secretion of androgens by the adrenal glands in early life can be caused by a genetic defect. In female infants the result is a variety of masculinizing effects including clitoral enlargement. In many cases it becomes very difficult to decide on the sex of these children. Although externally they appear male, genetically they are

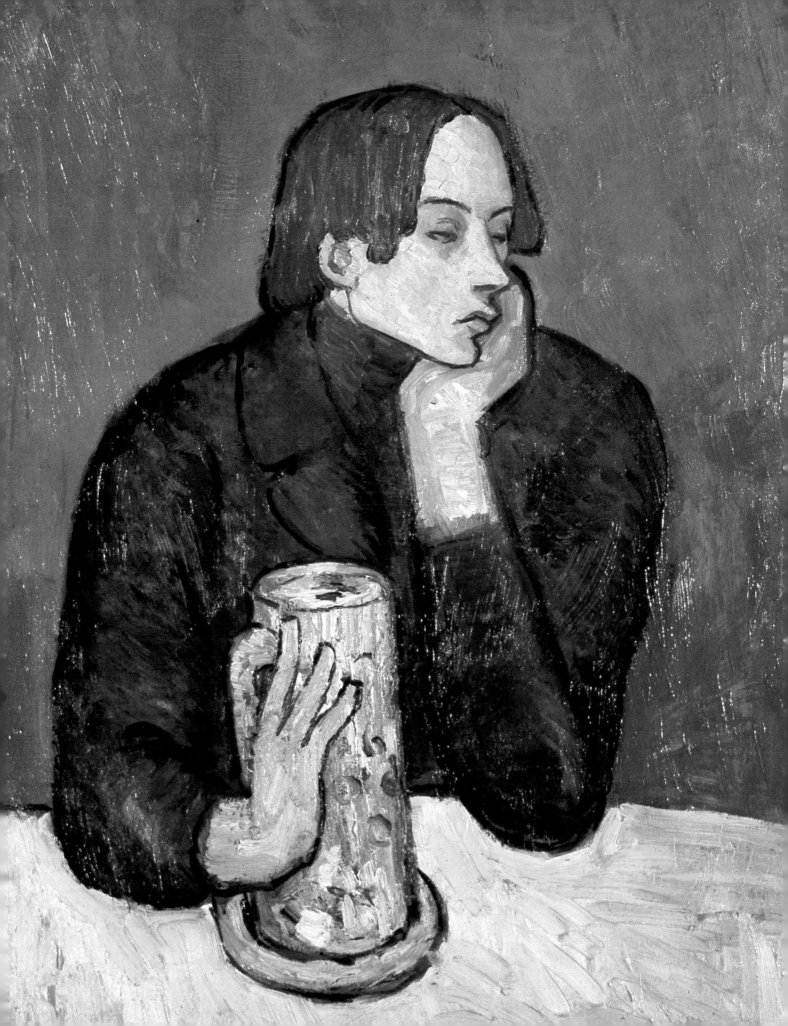

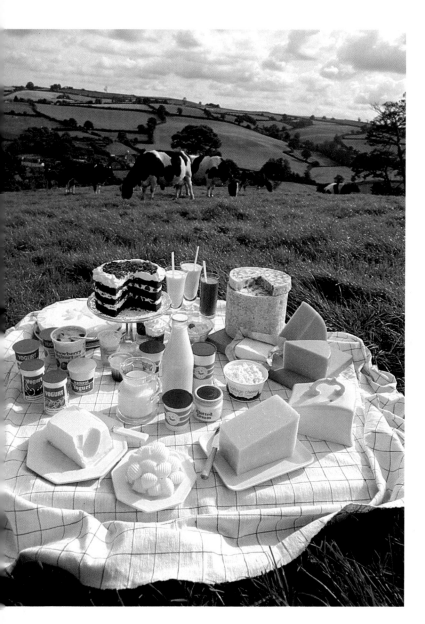

Dairy products such as milk, cream, yogurt and cheese are rich in calcium, and increasing the dietary intake of these foods is often sufficient treatment for hypoparathyroidism — undersecretion of parathormone by the parathyroid glands.

female. The condition may be caused by enzyme deficiencies which usually block the production of glucocorticoids and which subverts their precursors into the formation of androgens. Replacement of glucocorticoids prevents the overproduction of the male sex hormones. Ultimately they can become fertile and themselves bear children.

Another type of hormone closely related to those secreted by the adrenal cortex is represented by the anabolic steroids. These hormones cause increases in muscle bulk and, although banned by athletics authorities, have been used by athletes as part of their training programs. They remain, however, widely used and will probably continue to be so unless routine blood and urine tests are carried out on all competing athletes.

The adrenal medulla, the inner part of the gland, is both structurally and functionally distinct from the outer cortex. Its two hormones epinephrine and norepinephrine are secreted at times of either emotional or physical stress and increase the heart rate and force of beating. In addition the blood pressure rises, and blood is shunted away from nonessential sites such as the skin (which explains why stress results in cold clammy hands) to other parts of the body, such as muscles, which have to go into action to respond to any threat. Tumors of the adrenal medulla, called pheochromocytomas, may be present in either childhood or adulthood. Those in children are generally extremely malignant, and spread rapidly.

The Gonads: Testes or Ovaries

The ovaries are two almond-shaped organs approximately one-and-three-quarter inches long, situated within the pelvic girdle. Dispersed within each are collections of cells called follicles. At the center of each follicle is an ovum (or egg). During the first half of each menstrual cycle one follicle becomes the dominant one and undergoes full development and becomes a Graafian follicle, which secretes estrogen. Among other functions, estrogen prepares the lining of the womb to accept an ovum if it is fertilized.

During the second half of the menstrual cycle, after the ovum has been released, the follicle starts to secrete progesterone. The follicle at this stage is called the corpus luteum. If fertilization has not

Former President John F. Kennedy suffered from Addison's disease—undersecretion of adrenal hormones caused by atrophy of the adrenals. This condition can be treated with glucocorticoids.

taken place within 48 hours of the ovum's release, the ovum dies and the secretion of progesterone decreases from the seventh to fourteenth day after ovulation. Because its hormonal support has been withdrawn, the womb lining is eventually shed (as the menstrual "bleed"), and the cycle starts over again. All the hormonal changes are under the control of the gonadotropins secreted by the pituitary. Follicle-stimulating hormone has the dominant effect during the first half of the cycle and, as its name indicates, causes maturation of the follicle.

Just before ovulation there is a surge in the secretion of luteinizing hormone which both provokes ovulation and stimulates the corpus luteum to secrete progesterone. One of the most effective ways in which oral contraceptive pills work is by blocking the secretion of luteinizing hormone.

In humans this reproductive cycle occurs once every twenty-eight days. (In domestic or wild animals the reproductive urge is absent for most of the year, and only at certain times does the female come into heat, or "estrus," and permit a male to mate with her. In the case of some polar animals this happens only once a year; in mice, alternatively, it occurs every few days.) The American anatomist Edgar Allen was the first person to show that by removing the ovaries the cycle of changes in the womb and cervix could be abolished. In 1923 working together with his biochemist colleague, Edward Doisy, he collected large quantities of follicular fluid from the ovaries of female hogs. Purified, and injected into animals which had their ovaries removed, it was shown to produce the changes associated with the menstrual cycle. This work later led to the purification of estrogen.

The testes, like the ovaries, contain cells carrying genetic information for procreation (sperm) and other cells that secrete hormones (testosterone and androsterone). The male sex hormones are produced by small clusters of cells called Leydig cells.

Estrogens, progesterone, testosterone and androsterone are produced by both males and females. It is therefore essentially a difference in the relative production of the two types of hormones that governs male and female characteristics. Testosterone and androsterone bring about development of a beard and larger muscles, deepening of the voice and the maturation of the male genitalia. Estrogens and progesterone cause not only the changes associated with the menstrual cycle but also the characteristic female development of the breasts and hips.

Many disorders can affect the ovaries and testes.

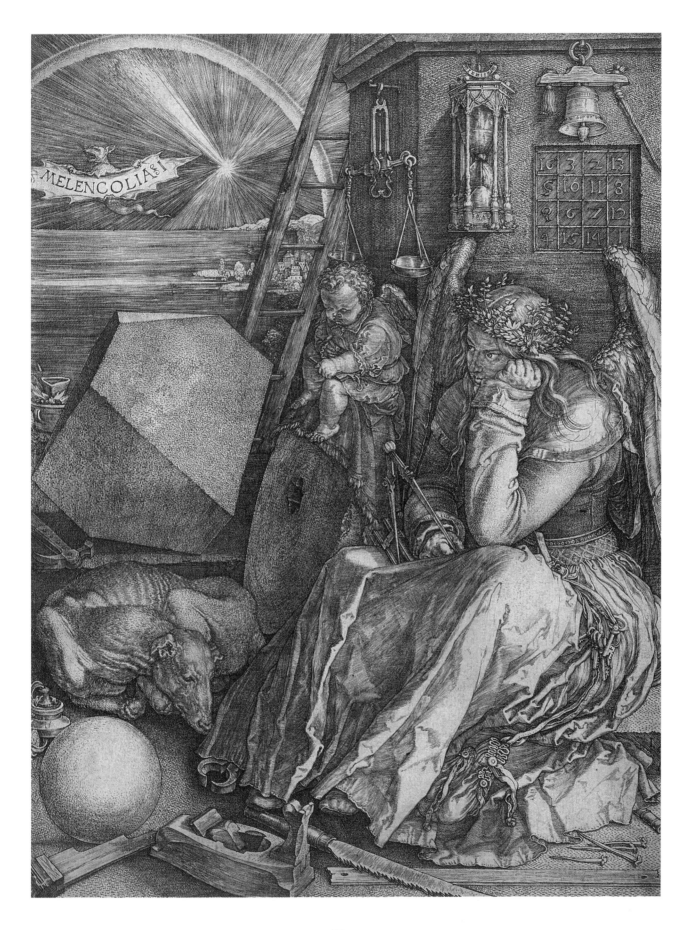

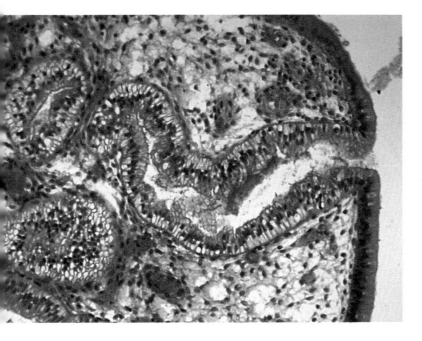

The testes are located outside the body because the lower temperatures there assist in the development of sperm. Yet the testes' own development starts high within the abdominal cavity and only at about the time of birth do they come to lie within the scrotum. In some cases, however, the testes either fail to descend or find their way into an abnormal site — the top of the thigh, for example — a condition termed cryptorchidism. Because the production of the male sex hormones is not affected by the higher temperatures of the body cavity, these people appear as normal males (although probably sterile). The best treatment for a case of undescended testicles in a boy aged less than three is surgery to restore the testes to their normal site in the hope that fertility may follow puberty.

Either males or females may undergo premature sexual development if for one reason or another the sex hormones are produced before the normal time. Some conditions may cause the normal changes of puberty to occur early, or a tumor may secrete either gonadotropins (usually because of some cerebral lesion) or sex hormones (usually through the gonads or adrenals) themselves. In addition to their precocious development of the secondary sexual characteristics these children grow more rapidly than normal. Such growth does not continue, however, and once the growth spurt is over the children are left shorter than normal because of the premature closure of the growth plates in the bones. In some cases these children are fertile. An extreme example is of a five-year-old Peruvian girl who gave birth in 1939.

The treatment of this condition depends on its cause. For example, if the sex hormones are being produced by a tumor, surgical intervention is essential. In contrast, the onset of puberty may sometimes be delayed. Most often, such a delay is simply part of normal variation. A delay in the onset of menstruation until a girl has reached the age of sixteen requires no medical investigation. There are, however, a number of potential causes for a delay in puberty in the female. These include mechanical obstruction to menstrual flow, failure of the endometrium to respond to hormonal stimulation, and ovarian or pituitary abnormalities. Tumors and other lesions may involve either the pituitary or the hypothalamus.

In the male the chief causes of delayed puberty are hypogonadism (testicular failure) and disorders which involve the pituitary and hypothalamus. Hypogonadism, whether affecting males or females, refers to some impairment of gonadal function. It may, for example, be associated with a genetic disorder which results in a defective gonad. In Turner's syndrome, a female instead of having two X chromosomes has only one; this is accompanied by multiple congenital abnormalities and a characteristically short stature with webbing of the neck and widely spaced nipples. Such females have small streaks of fibrous tissue instead of ovaries. Administration of estrogens can improve the external appearance of such females, but because they lack ova nothing can make them fertile. A genetic defect in males is Klinefelter's syndrome, in which the normal male complement of an X and Y chromosome is supplemented by an extra X chromosome. Men with this syndrome are tall and thin; their testes are small, and most often they are infertile.

Hypogonadism may be induced surgically. Removal of the gonads because of tumors within them or because of hormonal manipulation necessary for the treatment of certain tumors inevitably produces the condition. In the case of females,

Jonathan Swift's creations Gulliver and the Lilliputians (below), from the book Gulliver's Travels, illustrate a perennial fascination with extremes of human size. It is almost possible for the Lilliputians to have been a race of growth-hormone-deficient dwarfs, although in reality such dwarfism as this old engraving illustrates would not occur, because a lack of growth hormone from the pituitary gland (right) does not usually affect all the bones of the body equally, so some deformation or disfigurement occurs. Of all forms of dwarfism, hypopituitary dwarfs suffer from such malformations least, however.

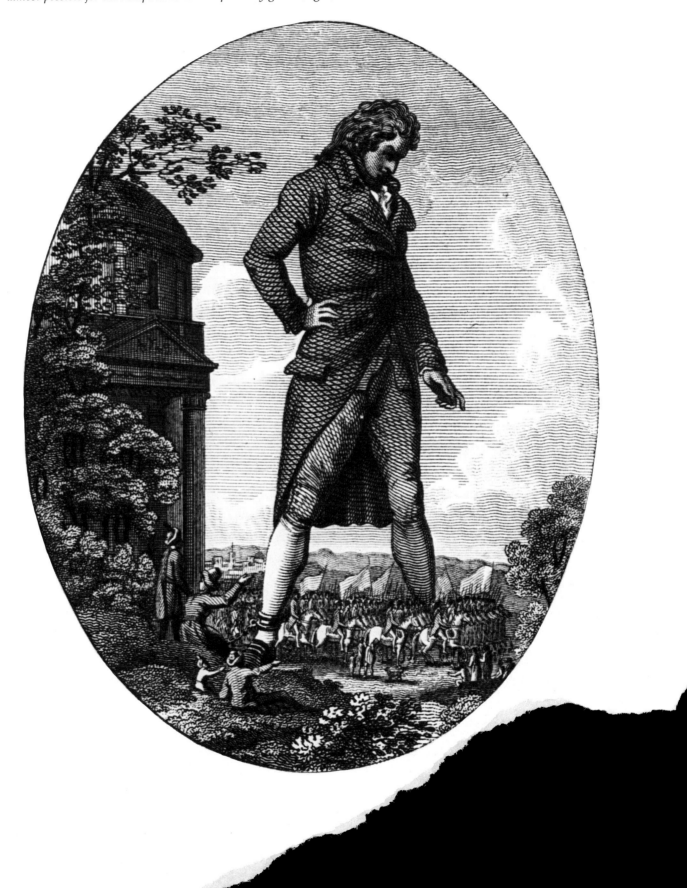

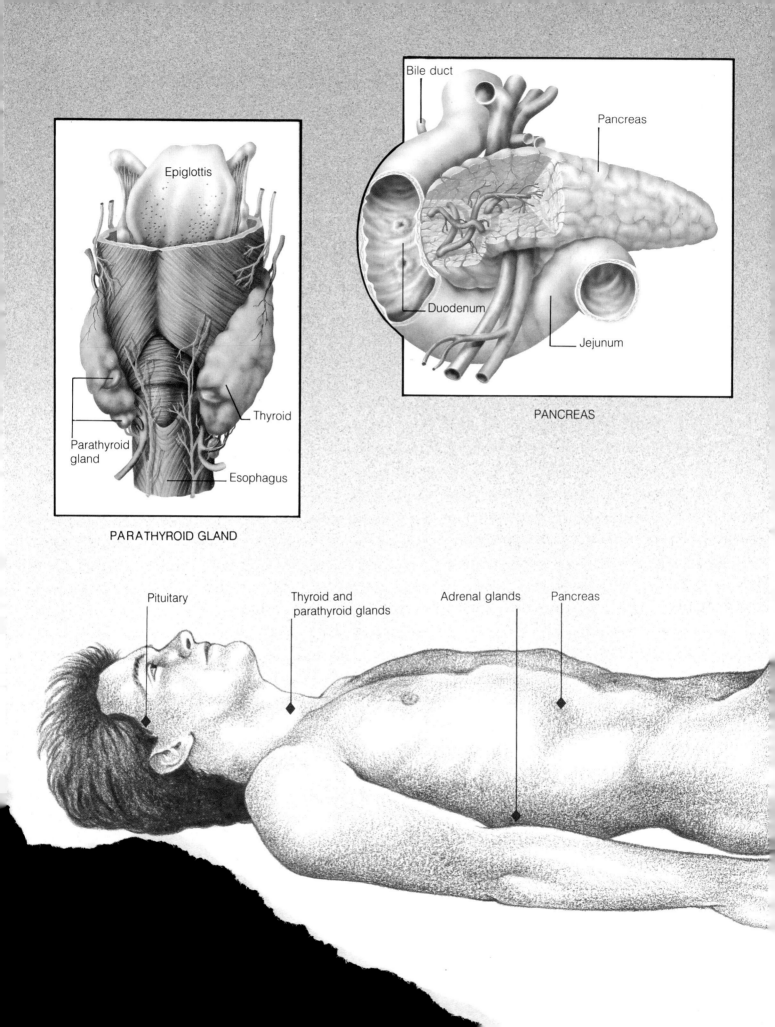

Epiglottis

Parathyroid gland

Thyroid

Esophagus

PARATHYROID GLAND

Bile duct

Pancreas

Duodenum

Jejunum

PANCREAS

Pituitary

Thyroid and parathyroid glands

Adrenal glands

Pancreas

The Endocrine Glands

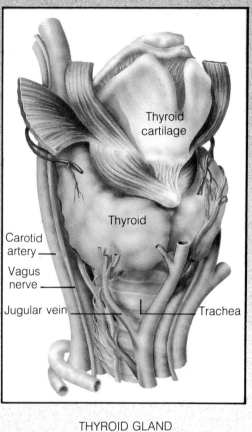

THYROID GLAND

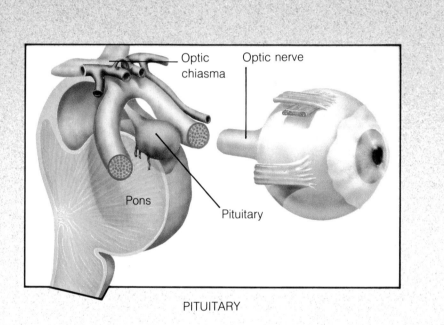

PITUITARY

The major hormones are secretions from the endocrine glands, which are sited at various locations within the body. Because hormones are carried in the bloodstream, each gland has veins and arteries connecting it with the circulatory system. The master gland, whose hormones control most of the other endocrine glands, is the pituitary, located in the center of the skull, in line with the bridge of the nose. The thyroid and parathyroids are in the neck, the thyroid in front around the larynx and the parathyroids at the back. There are two adrenal glands, one on top of each kidney, whose chief hormone – epinephrine – stimulates the body into action in times of danger. The pancreas, sited just below the liver, contains the Islets of Langerhans which secrete the hormone insulin. The metabolism of glucose, the sugar which fuels many of the body's internal processes, is controlled by the amount of insulin in the bloodstream. Sexual development and activity depends on sex hormones from the gonads, testes in a male and ovaries in a female.

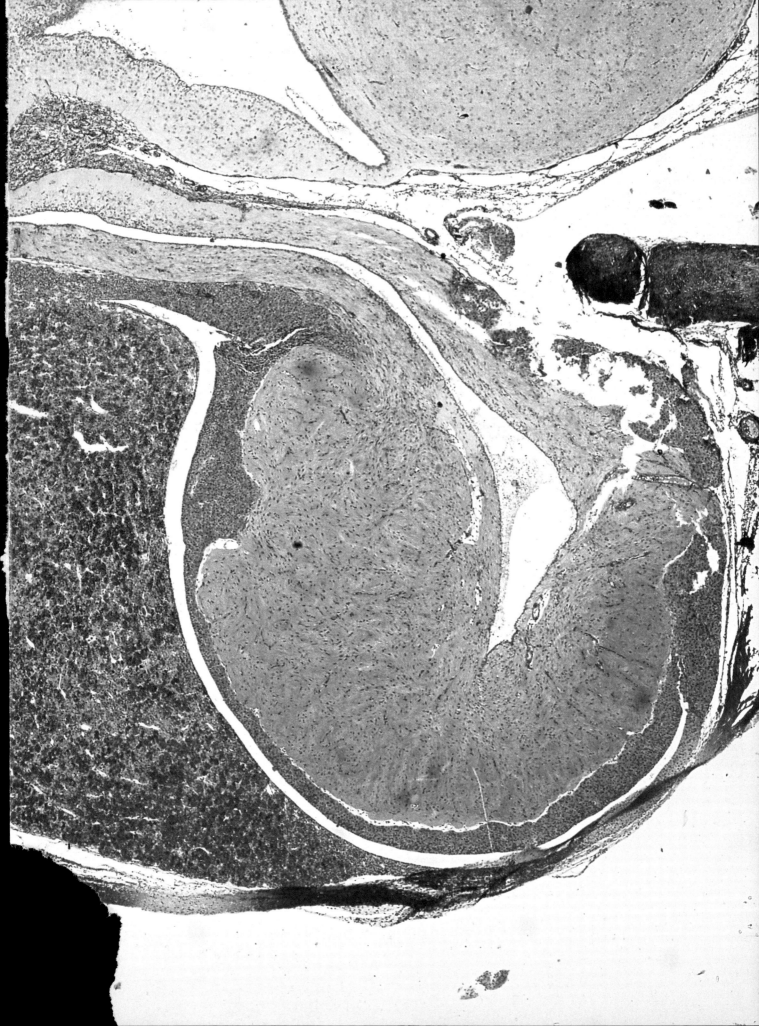

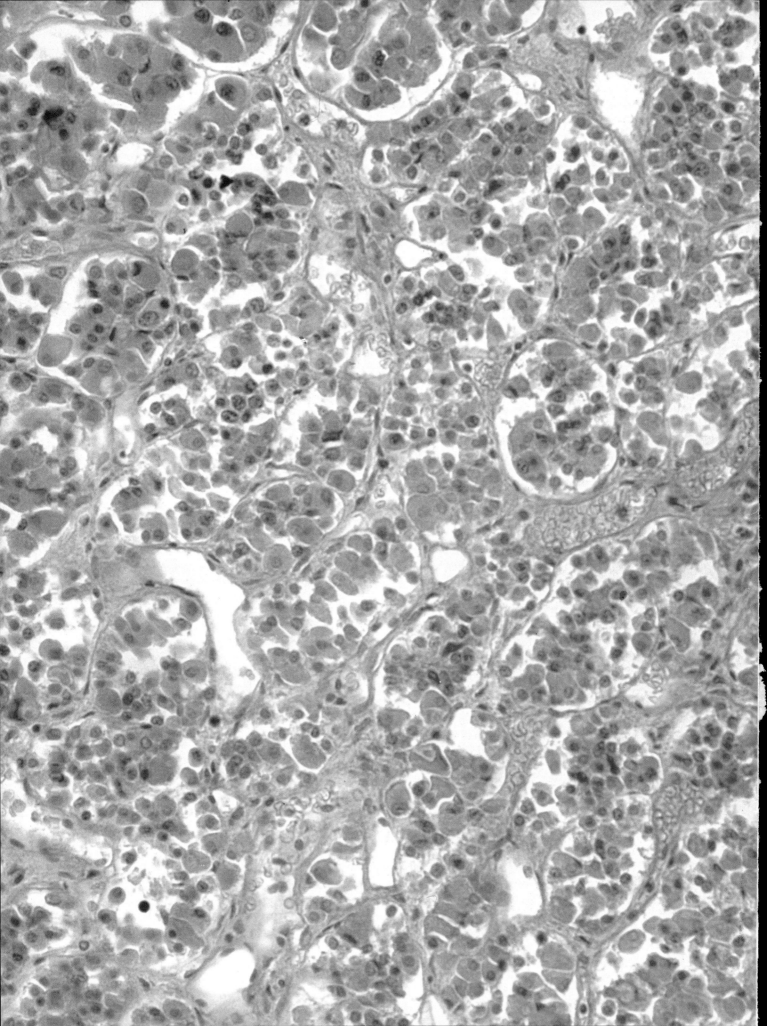

Female Sex Glands

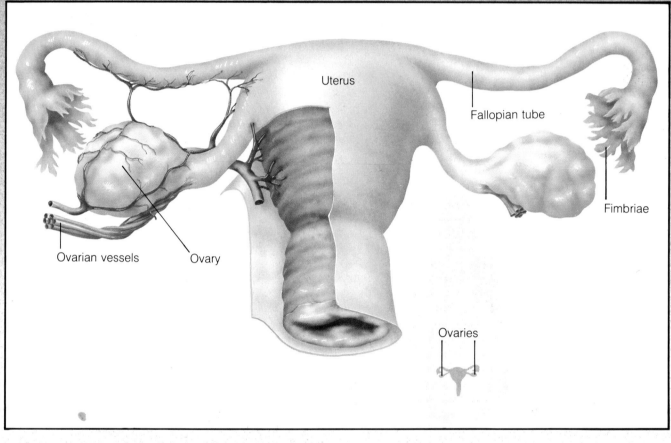

Uterus

Fallopian tube

Fimbriae

Ovarian vessels

Ovary

Ovaries

OVARIES

The female gonads are the ovaries, located on each side of the abdomen. Like the testes in males, they have a dual function. One is to produce and release ova (eggs), which they do about every twenty-eight days throughout a woman's childbearing life. At ovulation, an egg is released and caught up by the feathery fimbriae at the funnel-shaped entrance to the Fallopian tube. The egg then travels along the tube to the uterus. The other function of the ovaries is to secrete female sex hormones, such as estrogen and progesterone. These hormones are responsible for the development of secondary sexual characteristics in girls after puberty and, with others, are also responsible for the regular bodily changes that accompany the menstrual cycle. Egg release and hormone production cease at the menopause.

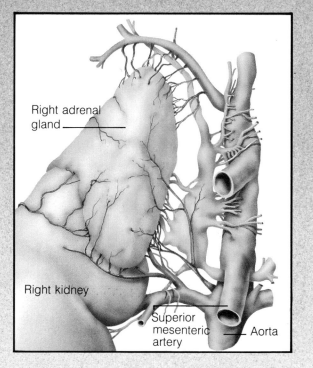

ADRENAL GLAND

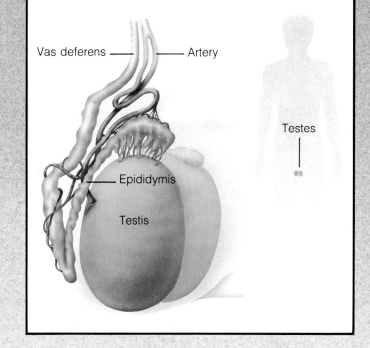

TESTES

The testes are located in the scrotum. In addition to producing sperm, they secrete testosterone. This male sex hormone is responsible for the development of secondary sexual characteristics in boys after puberty and for maintaining maleness throughout a man's adult life.

In Alice's Adventures in
Wonderland, *Alice ate a cake
labeled "Eat Me" or drank from a
bottle labeled "Drink Me" to grow*

*or shrink. The effects of growth
hormone, however — from pituitary
tissue (left) — are normally only
very gradual.*

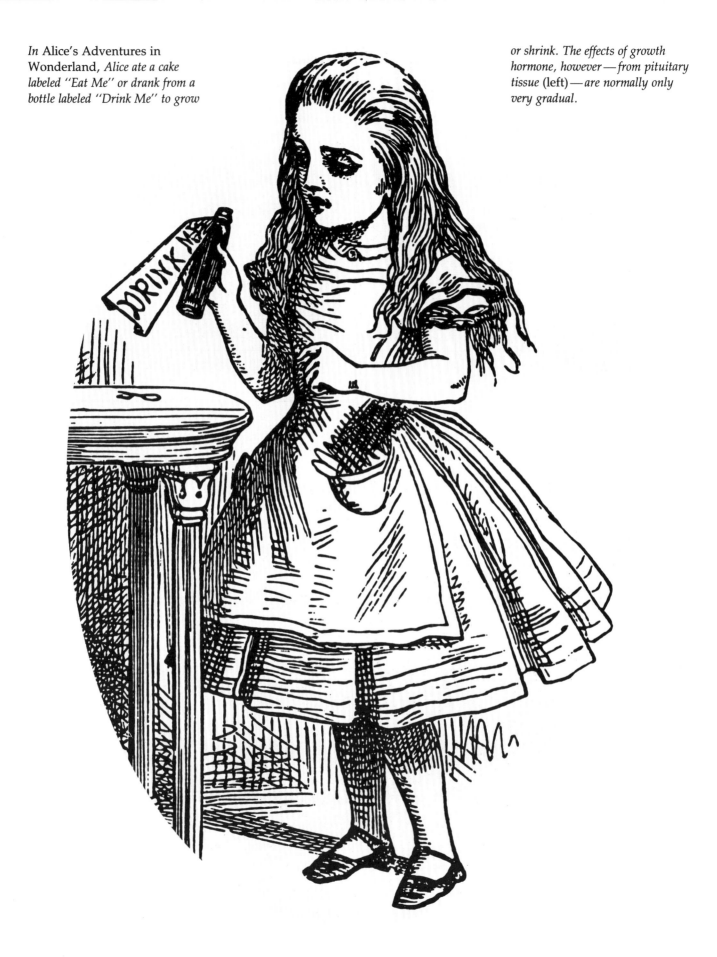

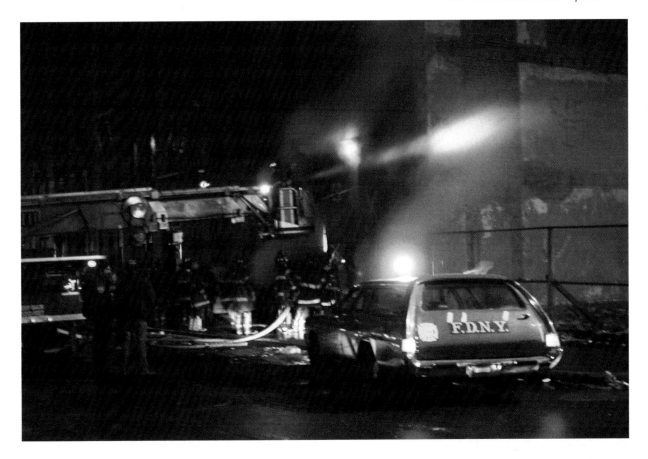

removal of the gonads results in a premature menopause or "change of life," which in some cases can be delayed by hormone replacement therapy. Naturally, the menopause is itself associated with a condition of hypogonadism.

The appearance of external sexual characteristics is determined by the relative levels of male and female sex hormones, but is not always strictly in accord with the genetic sex of an individual. Tests used at the Olympic Games to determine the sex of competitors rely on the fact that females have two X chromosomes whereas males have one X and one Y chromosome. A genetic female's second X chromosome, termed the Barr body, is visible in the nuclei of certain cells, most conveniently those lining the mouth.

If, within a genetic male, there is inadequate secretion of male sex hormones and a predominance of estrogens, it is possible for him to have the external appearance of a female. Such a condition is referred to as pseudohermaphroditism because the male only appears female but actually retains the genetic makeup and gonads (the testes) of the male. Female pseudohermaphrodites are perhaps more common; their external male appearance is due to excess production of androgens.

These conditions should be clearly distinguished from that of true hermaphrodites, who possess both ovaries and testes. Although true hermaphrodites are common in the animal kingdom and constitute the normal form of some, including earthworms and certain lizards, they are exceptionally rare among humans.

Several types of tumors can arise either in the ovaries or the testes, differing widely in their ability to spread within the patient. In fact most ovarian tumors are quite benign, or curable by simple surgical removal.

Gynecomastia is the development of breast tissue in a male; it is relatively common in all pubertal

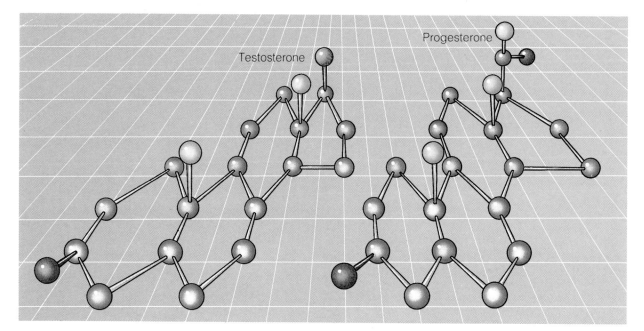

males, but it usually disappears. There are, however, a number of diseases that may produce gynecomastia, including alcoholic liver disease and hormone-secreting tumors; some drugs also cause this condition.

Other Endocrine Tissues

In addition to the ordinarily recognized endocrine glands there are cells scattered throughout the body which are endocrine in function, particularly in the gastrointestinal tract, where they are present in all areas but especially in the stomach and small intestine. Part of the difficulty in identifying these endocrine cells is that they are scattered individually among all the other cells of the bowel. In fact, the first hormone to be identified came from the small intestine: secretin — which stimulates water secretion by the pancreas — was identified at the turn of the century by two English physiologists, William Bayliss and Ernest Starling. The attention of endocrinologists then turned, for various reasons, to other organs, and it has only been in comparatively recent times that attention has again focused on this part of the body.

A large number of hormonal products have now been identified. These include gastrin (which increases the amount of acid produced by the stomach), cholecystokinin (which produces contraction of the gall bladder), pancreozymin (which stimulates enzyme secretion by the pancreas and has the same structure as cholecystokinin) and enteroglucagon (which also has properties similar to cholecystokinin). Several of these hormones have very similar structures, although they have different properties. Changes in the blood levels of all these hormones are brought about by the needs of the body during different stages of digestion. High levels of these hormones, however, may lead to disorders, especially gastrin which may cause duodenal ulceration.

The kidney is not normally thought of as an endocrine organ. Its major function is excretion of fluids, minerals and waste products. Despite this the kidney serves a number of important endocrine functions. It secretes the substance renin, which is important in controlling blood pressure. In 1939 the American physician Harry Goldblatt discovered that by partly clamping the arteries supplying the kidneys of a dog so as to reduce, but not halt, the blood flow to them, he could raise the animal's blood pressure. Furthermore, if he unclamped them the blood pressure returned to normal. He thought that the kidneys did this by secreting a substance which he called renin.

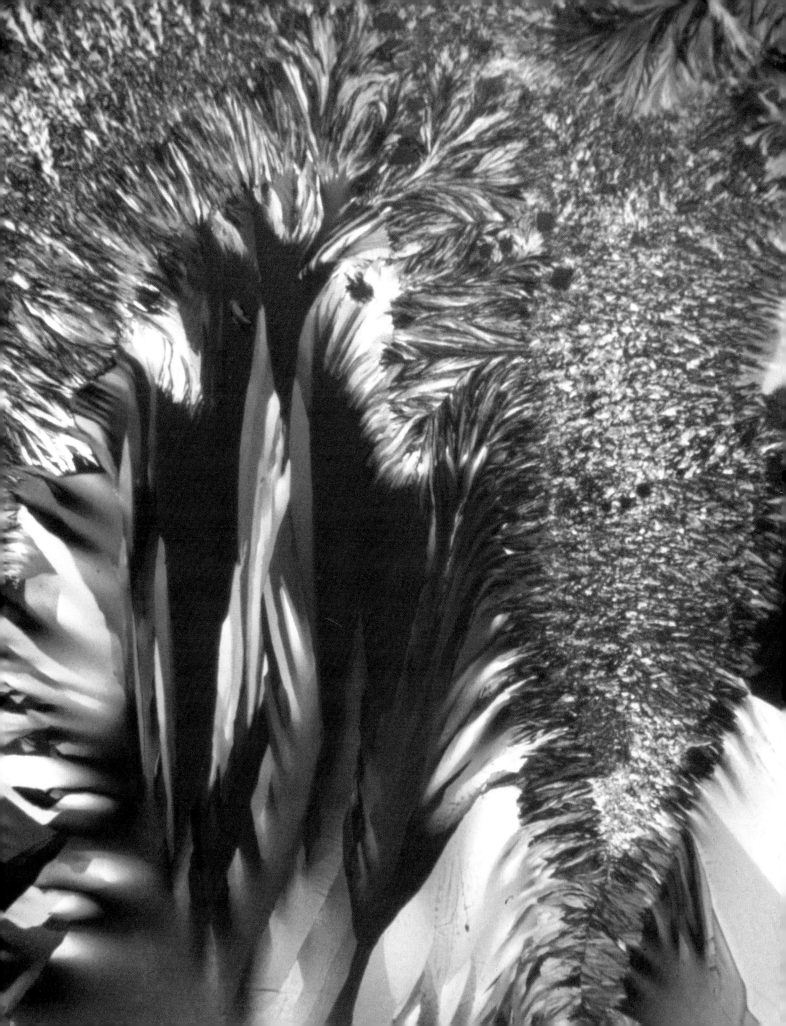

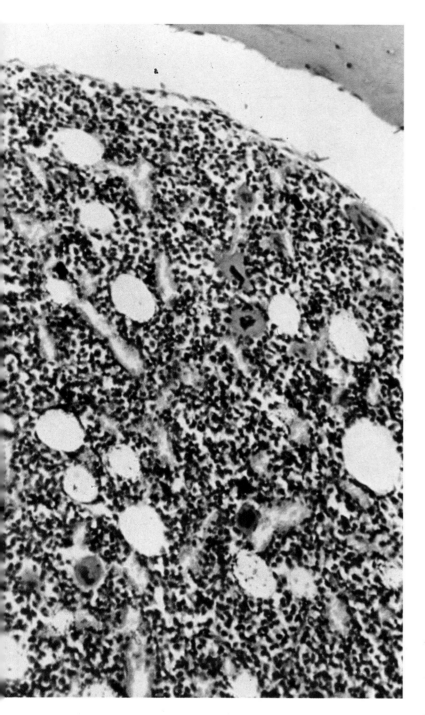

Red bone marrow—a section through which is shown in this photomicrograph—is stimulated by erythropoietin to produce red blood cells. This hormone is produced by the kidneys and is released in greater than normal amounts after bleeding, to make good the resultant red cell deficit.

Curiously, renin had been isolated from the kidney in 1898 but its function had remained unknown for forty years. It is now known that renin does not raise the blood pressure directly. Instead it acts as an enzyme to start a reaction to break down a protein present in the blood to form angiotensin. This causes direct constriction of blood vessels and stimulates the release of aldosterone from the adrenal cortex, thereby producing a rise in blood pressure. The structure of angiotensin was determined by Professor W. S. Pearl in London and was the first protein hormone of which the complete structure was understood.

Another hormonal substance produced by the kidney is erythropoietin, which is crucial in stimulating the production of red blood cells by the bone marrow. If, for any reason, there is loss of blood from the body, erythropoietin is produced to help make good the deficit. When a patient has cancer of the kidney, excess erythropoietin may be produced, stimulating an overproduction of red cells, and the blood becomes so viscous that its flow through the body is slowed down.

During pregnancy the placenta develops and sends tongues of tissue into the endometrial lining of the womb. Derived almost entirely from fetal tissues, its function is to allow the maternal circulation to provide essential nutrients to the fetus and to remove unwanted waste products. In addition, the placenta is responsible for secreting an impressive array of hormones which sustain the fetus during pregnancy and prepare the mother's body for breast-feeding. These include human chorionic gonadotropin (HCG), which stimulates the corpus luteum to produce progesterone until such time as the placenta itself takes over that function. Other sex steroids secreted by the placenta include estrogens and androgens. Some of these, together with another hormone, human chorionic somatomammotropin, cause development of the breast in preparation for lactation. Several other hormones (including renin) are produced by the placenta, although their function remains unclear.

The Pineal Gland

Named for its pine-cone shape, the pineal gland is even smaller than the pituitary. It is made up of

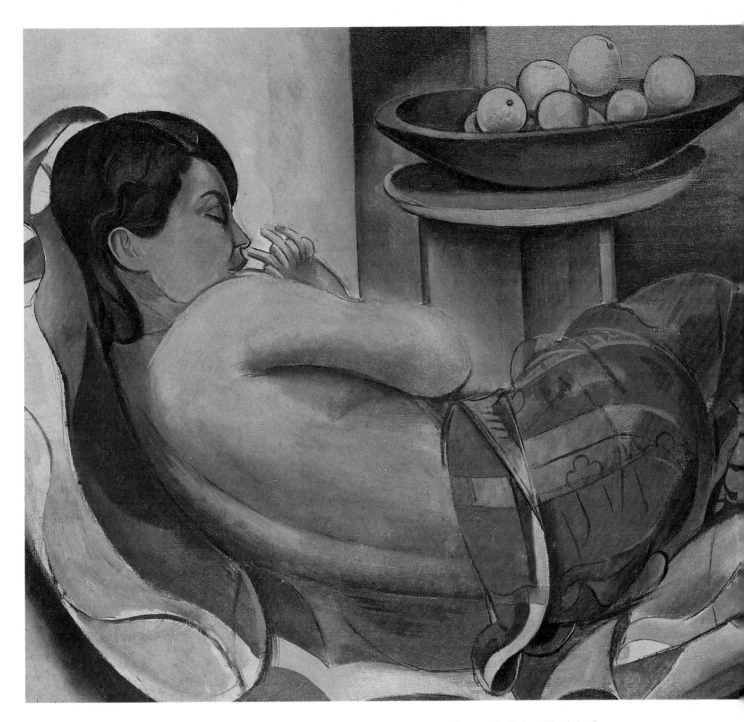

Sleep can be induced by injecting melatonin, one of the hormones secreted by the pineal gland. The level of this substance in the blood varies on a 24-hour cycle, being higher at night than during daylight hours. For this reason scientists believe that it may be involved in controlling the sleep cycle.

Earthworms, here shown mating, are naturally true hermaphrodites, a condition that is abnormal — and extremely rare — in humans. Pseudohermaphroditism, the external appearance of one sex but the genetic makeup and reproductive organs of the other, is more common. In males it is usually caused by a deficiency of male sex hormones before birth. In females it results from excess male sex hormones before or after birth.

The various glands of the endocrine system secrete many different hormones, each of which has a specific effect. The principal hormones and their main effects are summarized in the diagram (right).

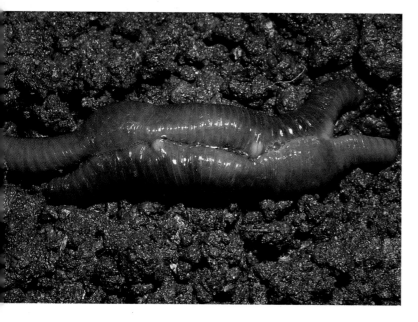

peculiar cells with properties somewhere between those of nerve cells and epithelial cells. Attached to the base of the brain, its inaccessibility partially accounts for the ignorance of its function. It secretes a large number of active chemicals, the most important of which is melatonin, a substance present in higher concentrations in the blood during the night. An injection of melatonin induces sleepiness; it is therefore possible that it plays an important role in controlling the sleep cycle. Melatonin also inhibits the secretion of gonadotropins. It is for this reason that tumors of the pineal may slow down the development of sexual maturity or in some cases accelerate it.

In creatures such as the frog, melatonin has a profound effect on pigmentation: by responding to light in a way that is not fully understood, the pineal gland modifies the frog's skin color. The relatively large pineal located just behind the bones of the human forehead led some ancient observers to consider that the pineal gland was in fact a "third eye." The observations described above lend some support to this concept.

The Thymus

For a long time scientists knew little about the thymus gland, but it is now known to be central to the body's defense mechanisms. Lymphocytes, a type of white blood cell, mature in the thymus before becoming fully able to help rid the body of certain infectious agents such as viruses and cancerous cells. How the thymus helps in the development of lymphocytes remains obscure, but it is known that the thymus produces a number of hormonelike substances, such as thymusin, which do appear to stimulate this process. In this way the thymus can be considered — at least in part — as an endocrine gland.

The thymus is located just behind the breastbone, and reaches its maximum size relative to the rest of the body at birth, when it is the size of the baby's fist. Later it shrinks progressively with increasing age. This relentless decrease in size may be one reason that infections are relatively common in older people.

Abnormalities of the thymus indicate the importance of its normal activity. For example, children born without one are prone to life-threatening infections. David, the "Bubble Boy," lived in an isolated protected plastic "bubble" environment for about ten years to protect him from infection. Patients with thymic tumors (thymomas) are susceptible to a wide range of infections, bacterial, viral and fungal, and may become anemic. Yet in an adult of ordinary health, the absence of a thymus through surgery may make little difference. Tumors, however, are also associated with a range of so-called autoimmune diseases, characterized by the body's defense system attacking parts of itself. One of the most common autoimmune disorders associated with thymic tumors is myasthenia gravis, a condition characterized by the progressive paralysis of the muscles.

In some cases, removal of a thymic tumor leads to dramatic improvement in the patient's condition. Some years ago it was suggested that crib deaths, sudden deaths occurring in apparently fit infants (the Sudden Infant Death Syndrome), were due to a generalized enlargement of the lymphoid tissue of the body, including the thymus. This even led to perfectly normal thymuses in young children being irradiated to reduce their size. Today it is felt that this enlargement is of no importance in itself. In some cases, however, the enlargement may be due to a viral infection which may be of significance in some of these deaths.

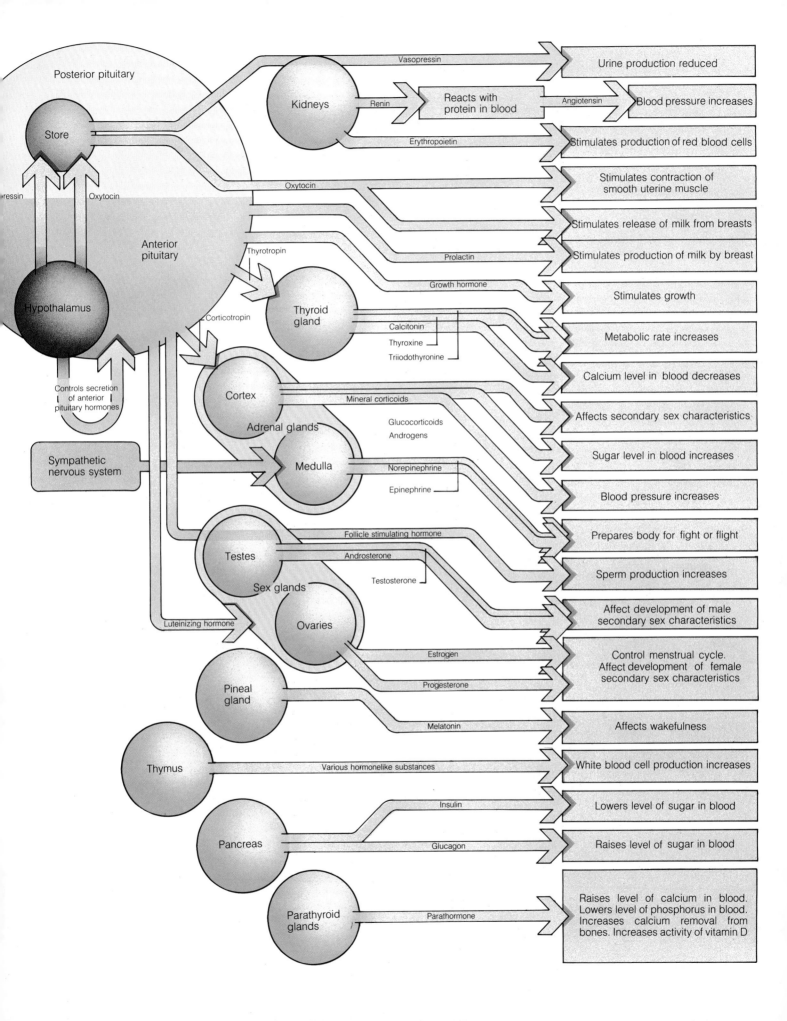

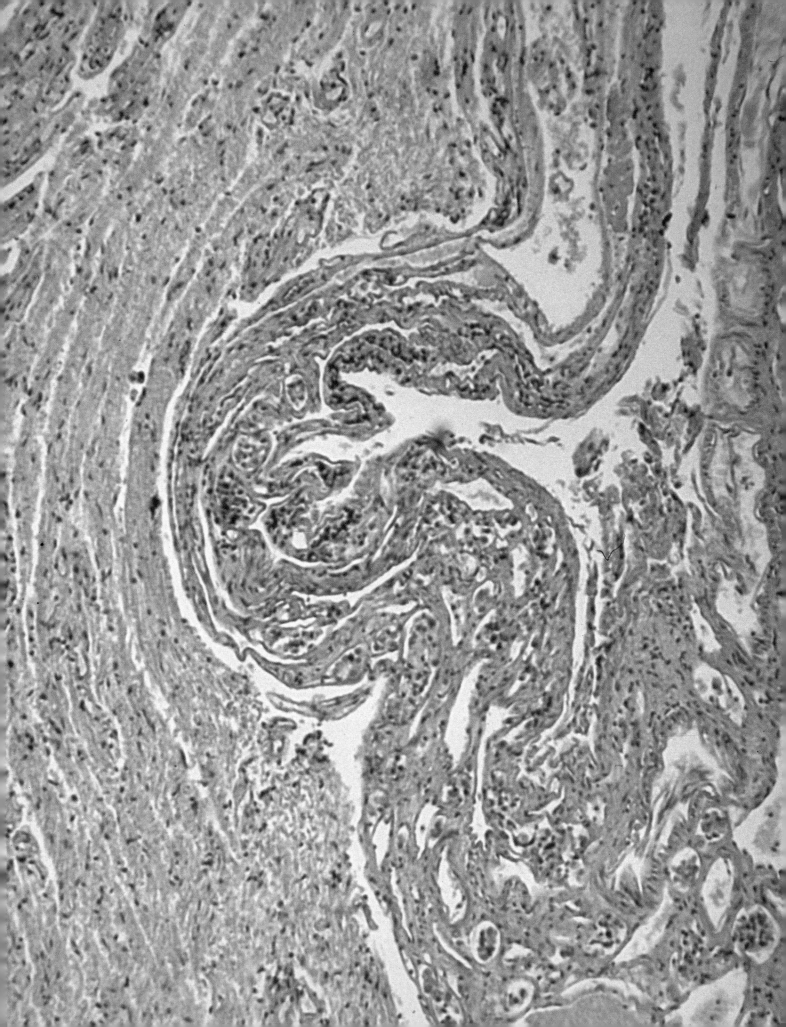

Chapter 3

The Chemical Conductor

The pituitary gland, which hangs from the base of the brain by a short stalk, lies within a small cavity of the sphenoid bone, just above the roof of the mouth. It is made up of two lobes, but it is no bigger than a pea and weighs about one-fiftieth of an ounce. Yet this tiny structure controls many of the hormone secretions of the endocrine glands dispersed throughout the body. Indeed, it has been described as "the conductor of the endocrine orchestra," and its intimate connection with the brain allows the two communicating systems of the body — nerves and hormones — to interact.

Early ideas about the function of the pituitary gland were voiced as far back as in the Greco-Roman period. Galen (A.D. 130–200), who was probably the greatest medical man of antiquity after Hippocrates, speculated that "animal spirit" was formed from "vital spirit" in the brain, and that the waste products of this reaction flowed down to the base of the brain, through the pituitary stalk and into the gland itself. From this "phlegmatic glandule" the waste products passed through the sphenoid bone and into the nose, where they were excreted as "pituita" or nasal mucus.

Many seventeenth-century anatomists disputed Galen's theory but were unable to do more than speculate upon the function of the pituitary gland. Indeed, the gland seemed to attract little interest until the end of the eighteenth and beginning of the nineteenth century, when many physicians thought that it was an enlarged ganglion representing the head of the sympathetic nervous system. It was believed to be concerned with body movements and balance, and to have an important function in "creative intellectual activity." In 1838 the German anatomist Martin Rathke described the development of the pituitary gland and showed that the anterior (and intermediate) lobe of the gland originated through growth upward from the roof of the mouth, whereas the posterior lobe was

The pituitary gland, shown here in cross section, is the second-in-command of the hormonal system, receiving its orders from the hypothalamus and delegating its hormones in turn to carry out their functions. This pea-sized gland of tremendous importance is located just above the palate from where it coordinates the interaction of nerves and hormones.

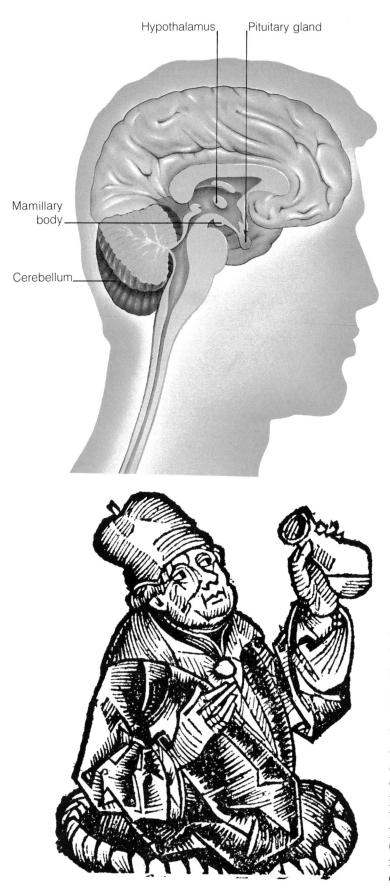

Hypothalamus　　Pituitary gland

Mamillary
body

Cerebellum

formed from a downward growth of nerves from the brain. The two lobes join to each other during fetal development.

The significance of this observation was not really appreciated at that time, yet contemporary historical descriptions of post-mortem examinations make it clear that an enlarged pituitary gland was, even then, associated with unexplained pathological conditions. This attribution, dating mainly from 1886, when the French neurologist Pierre Marie (1853–1940) published the first of his papers on acromegaly, was important in itself. The reason was that only through the knowledge of pituitary disease did the functions of the pituitary gland begin to be understood. Marie described a number of patients with very coarse facial features — a long face, prominent eyebrow ridges, a jutting jaw — and excessively large hands and feet. Of course he did not know what caused these abnormalities, but he noted that in all the cases there was a particularly enlarged pituitary gland —"the size of a hen's egg or even an apple."

Toward the end of the last century the experimentalists began to look at the effects of removing the pituitary gland. At the same time, more information was becoming available about the clinical symptoms associated with pathological conditions of the pituitary. One of the major technical advances during the first decade of the twentieth century was the ability to remove the pituitary gland through the nose (transphenoidal surgery). Previously the gland had been removed by cutting the skull, and lifting the front part of the brain — needless to say, the trauma accompanying that operation more often than not produced severe complications, if not actually resulting in death on the operating table.

In 1909 the American neurosurgeon Harvey Williams Cushing (1869–1939) summarized the current knowledge of the pituitary gland in an address to the American Medical Association. He concluded his talk by saying that there were two pathological conditions: one due to overactivity of the anterior lobe of the pituitary gland (hyperpituitarism), and the other due to underactivity (hypopituitarism). Cushing stated that the former manifests itself chiefly through a process of overgrowth — gigantism or acromegaly — and

58

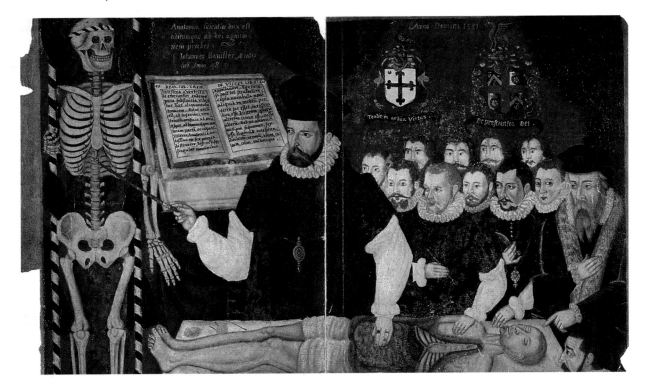

that the latter results in an excessive, often rapid, desposition of fat with persistence of infantile sexual characteristics or the loss of characteristics aquired in adolescence. In the same year Cushing successfully removed about one-third of the pituitary gland of an acromegalic patient; the patient was relieved of his condition and remained symptom-free for around twenty years afterward. Cushing remarked in a letter to his father that the pituitary "seems to be an important gland."

A year later, in 1910, Harvey Cushing and his collaborators provided the first evidence of a link between the anterior lobe of the pituitary gland and the reproductive organs. It was not, however, until 1932 and the latter part of his career that he associated overactivity of the pituitary gland with excessive secretions of the adrenal cortex. The condition, Cushing's syndrome, was named for him, although it is perhaps unfortunate that he is best remembered for that rather than for his earlier astute experimental work, which gave important insights into the functions and influence of the pituitary gland.

During the first fifteen years of the twentieth century, knowledge about the posterior pituitary gland was also increasing. In Edinburgh, Scotland, Sir Edward Sharpey-Schafer and his colleagues studied the effects of posterior pituitary extracts, showing that they had blood-pressure-raising actions and inhibited urine flow. In 1911, scientists in Philadelphia described a substance in the posterior pituitary that controlled the release of milk from women's breasts after childbirth. By 1912 others had made the connection between a malfunction of posterior pituitary secretions and diabetes insipidus — a syndrome characterized by the uncontrolled production of urine and an intense thirst.

Within the first three decades of this century the major functions of the pituitary gland became known. This was mainly achieved by studying the effects of removing the pituitary gland (hypophysectomy) and treating hypophysectomized animals with pituitary extracts. A few historical landmarks deserve mention. In 1912 it was demonstrated that the adrenal glands shrink after hypophysectomy. Twelve years later it was reported that this effect could be prevented by the

Harvey Cushing

The Patient's Friend

If he had not been a neurosurgeon, Harvey Williams Cushing could have been an equally successful historian. History was one of his major interests and—because he was a medical man himself—medical history was his specialty. Few, if any, other surgeons have won a Pulitzer Prize for (medical) biography, as he did. Yet he is much better known for his gradual devising of new techniques in difficult neurosurgical operations, and his definition and explanation of the chronic wasting disease now called Cushing's syndrome.

Cushing was born into a family of physicians in Cleveland, Ohio, in April 1869. Although he studied medicine at Yale College, it was from Harvard Medical School that he graduated in 1895. The next four years, formative for him, were spent in practical training in Boston and Baltimore, some of the time under the aegis of the celebrated surgical innovator William Halsted. He then spent a further period of instruction in Switzerland and England, before returning to Johns Hopkins University. In Switzerland he was taught by the great Theodor Kocher, who encouraged him to specialize in neurosurgery, and it was accordingly with Sir Charles

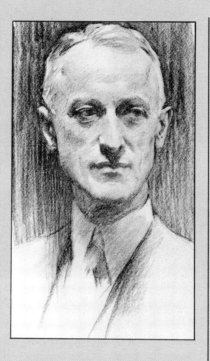

Sherrington, a leading neurophysiologist, that he studied in England.

Back in the USA he began investigating the functions and disorders of the pituitary gland, and inaugurated a series of experiments to discover how best to gain surgical access to this gland which, after all, is almost in the middle of the head. His energetic reforms of pre-operative investigation of the patients' case histories, his concern, and the number of cases of blindness caused by pressure on the optic nerve by pituitary tumors that he cured, all won him renown and admirers. His particular care

for patients' well-being is illustrated by the fact that although he was a neurosurgeon, he devised new systems for the control of bleeding and also of blood pressure during surgical operations.

In 1912, becoming nationally known for his successful techniques in neurosurgery, Cushing was appointed Professor of Surgery at the Harvard Medical School and Surgeon-in-Chief at the Peter Bent Brigham Hospital in Boston. Within a couple of years, however, the events of World War I overtook him, and he was enlisted in the Army Medical Corps. At the end of the war he was created Senior Consultant in Neurological Surgery to the American Expeditionary Force. Meanwhile, in 1917, he had published what came to be seen as a definitive account of tumors of the acoustic nerves.

Cushing went on to explain several more of the dysfunctions of pituitary secretion, such as acromegaly and hypopituitary dwarfism. His account of what came to be called Cushing's syndrome was, however, later found to be slightly inaccurate.

Appointed Sterling Professor of Neurology at Yale University in 1933, he retired in 1937 and died in October 1939.

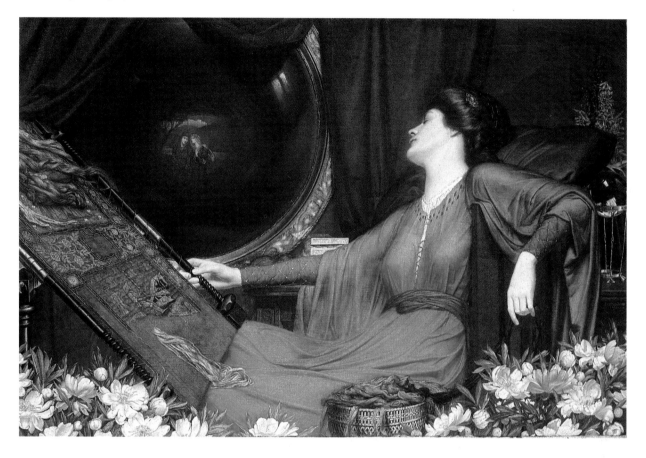

administration of pituitary extracts, although by that time it had already been shown that body growth in the young could be stimulated by giving injections of anterior lobe extracts. And within another three years, in 1927, the activity of the ovaries and testes was proved to be maintained by secretions from the anterior pituitary. Furthermore, it was confirmed that the thyroid gland was also under the control of the anterior pituitary.

So by the end of the 1930s it was known that the anterior pituitary gland regulated the hormones of the ovary and testis, the adrenal cortex, and the thyroid gland; it was known also to release a substance which promoted growth. The next step in the story was the identification of the hormones themselves.

In 1927 the German gynecologists Selmar Aschheim and Bernhardt Zondek reported that there were probably two hormones that controlled the gonads; they called them prolan A and prolan B. The notion of two hormones was strongly contested at the time, although the two scientists' insights were proved correct: there are indeed two gonadotropins — luteinizing hormone (LH) and follicle-stimulating hormone (FSH). The discovery of the gonadotropins led Aschheim and Zondek to develop the first pregnancy test, which was published to the scientific community in 1928. They found that the urine of pregnant women contains an active principle similar to the gonadotropins. By injecting urine from a pregnant woman into a female frog, the frog's ovaries were stimulated to produce eggs. Thus if a sample of urine from a woman caused a frog to ovulate, then the woman who provided the sample was pregnant.

In the 1930s and 1940s, chemists and biochemists were actively trying to isolate the pituitary hormones in a pure form. Countless extractions and purifications were undertaken until finally minute quantities of a pure substance remained

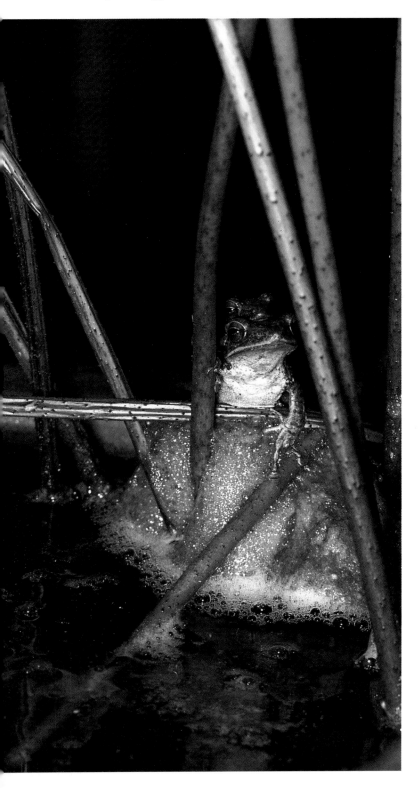

which was uncontaminated by other hormones or chemicals. The substance could then be analyzed so that chemists could discover the basic composition of the hormone molecule.

The Pituitary and Hypothalamus

Given that the pituitary secretes hormones some of which regulate the activity of other endocrine glands, what effect does its connection with the brain have, and how does the brain control the secretory activity of the gland? It was in the years between 1930 and 1950 that ideas about brain-pituitary interactions emerged, and scientists discovered how the hypothalamus (the area of the brain to which the pituitary is attached by its stalk) controls the hormone secretions emitted by the pituitary gland.

In the first decade of this century the famous Spanish histologist Ramón y Cajal described some "strange-looking" nerve cells whose axons projected to the posterior lobe of the pituitary gland. His observations were ignored at the time, but during the 1930s scientists studying the fine structure of the hypothalamus of fishes also observed unusual cells in this brain area. They found that the cells were full of small granules and looked more like the secretory type of cell than the usual type of neuron.

When more sohpisticated histological staining methods were developed, the axons of these secretory cells were seen to extend all the way down to the posterior pituitary, and it was also discovered that these neurons released the two posterior lobe hormones, oxytocin and vaso-pressin. So, for the first time, it was shown that nerve cells in the hypothalamus could synthesize and release hormones from their axon terminals into the blood circulation. These unique cells were in consequence called "neurosecretory cells," because they were neurons with a hormone-secreting function.

Later, it was discovered how the hormone secretions of the anterior lobe were controlled by the hypothalamus. In this case it was known that the hormones were not released from nerve endings because the anterior lobe contains very few nerve terminals, and is largely composed of non-neural secretory cells.

In 1930 scientists first described the network of

When the hypothalamus receives a message from the brain it releases hormones from neurosecretory cells. Some of these hormones are intended for storage and travel along the neurosecretory tracts to the posterior pituitary—they include oxytocin and vasopressin. Most hormones, however, are released for immediate action from the hypothalamus. They are carried to the anterior pituitary, where they stimulate the secretion of particular hormones. The six main hormones from this lobe of the pituitary are growth hormone, prolactin, luteinizing hormone, adrenocorticotropic hormone and follicle-stimulating hormone.

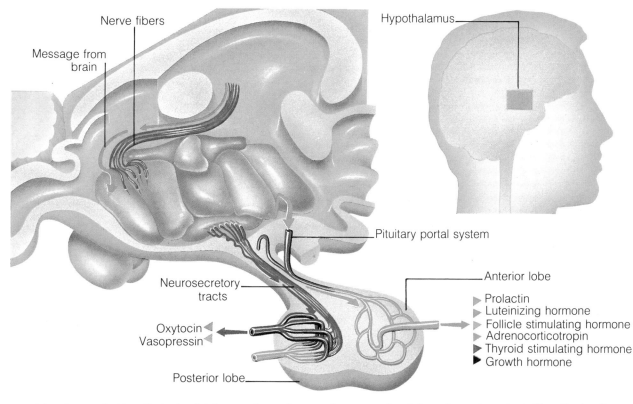

Nerve fibers

Message from brain

Hypothalamus

Pituitary portal system

Neurosecretory tracts

Anterior lobe
- Prolactin
- Luteinizing hormone
- Follicle stimulating hormone
- Adrenocorticotropin
- Thyroid stimulating hormone
- Growth hormone

Oxytocin
Vasopressin

Posterior lobe

fine blood vessels (capillaries) which runs from the base of the hypothalamus (an area called the median eminence) through the pituitary stalk and into the anterior lobe of the pituitary gland. Immediately afterward, ardent controversy sprang up about the direction of the blood flow in these hypophyseal (pituitary) portal capillaries. Was it from the hypothalamus to the pituitary or from the pituitary to the hypothalamus?

It was not until the early 1950s that the mechanism by which the hypothalamus controls anterior pituitary hormone secretions was finally elucidated. The credit for this must go to the work of the English endocrinologist Geoffrey W. Harris and his collaborators, who unequivocally showed that nerve cells in the hypothalamus release factors into the hypophyseal portal vessels. These factors are carried in the capillaries through which they reach the anterior lobe of the pituitary gland and stimulate or inhibit the release of hormones. Thus the anterior pituitary gland is controlled by specialized nerve cells (neurosecretory cells) in the hypothalamus which, unlike those associated with the posterior lobe, do not project directly to the gland but release their products into the local blood circulation — this is known as a "neurohumoral" control mechanism.

Extracts of hypothalamic tissue were shown to contain active substances which stimulated or inhibited the release of anterior pituitary hormones. During the 1960s, there was intensive research to identify these substances. Two independent American teams of physiologists, one headed by Andrew Victor Schally in New Orleans, the other by Roger Guillemin in La Jolla, California, came up with the first answer. But it had taken several years of arduous work, bitter rivalry between the two competing groups, and nearly a million dollars of research funds. Between 1964 and 1967 Guillemin's laboratory processed fifty tons of hypothalamic tissue from sheep (purchased at forty cents a hypothalamus); Schally was more fortunate — the meat packers Oscar Mayer & Co. donated one million pig hypothalamuses.

Nevertheless, by the mid-1960s, the financial backers of both teams were becoming impatient.

The hormone-secreting vesicles of a pituitary cell (below right), photographed using an electron microscope, are easier to see and quantify in the false-color computer-enhanced matrix (below left).

Stress (right) and cold *(bottom)* are conditions in which the endocrine and nervous systems come into play. Cold, for example, causes the thyroid gland to stimulate the body's metabolism and generate more heat.*

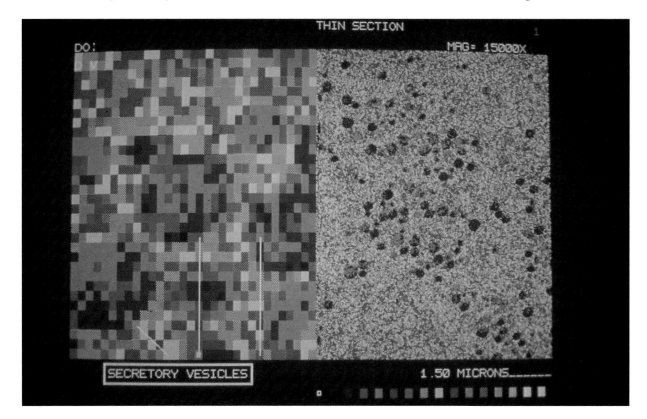

The interminable processing and extraction of brain tissue finally resulted in the two groups' publishing the identical structure of pig and sheep thyrotropin-releasing hormone in 1969. Both groups found the hormone to be a small peptide, made up of three amino acids (basic constituents of peptides and proteins), which stimulates the release of thyrotropin-stimulating hormone from the anterior pituitary.

The isolation of thyrotropin-releasing hormone (TRH) marked the end of the first lap of the race — to that point essentially a dead heat. Schally won the second lap in 1972 by discovering the structure of the releasing hormone which stimulates secretion of the gonadotropins; and Guillemin won the third in 1973, by isolating the hormone somatostatin, which inhibits the release of growth hormone. In 1977 they shared the Nobel Prize in physiology or medicine (along with Rosalyn Yalow for her radioimmunoassay technique) for their work on these hypothalamic releasing and inhibiting hormones. They could be

said to have arrived neck-and-neck at the finishing-post in Stockholm. Reasearch continued, and by the mid-1980s the releasing hormones for corticotropin and growth hormone had also been discovered.

In the functioning of the pituitary, the special nerve cells which secrete hormones are of enormous importance. In terms of pituitary activity, the neurosecretory cells can perhaps be regarded as transducers, which convert an electrical (neural) signal into a hormonal signal. These neurons can receive electrical impulses from many areas of the brain, and in this way information from divergent sources can be integrated and translated into a hormonal signal. For example, hormone secretions can be effected by changes in the external environment. If the body becomes very cold, it is thought that the hypothalamus switches on the activity of the thyroid glands, so that metabolic rate — and thus heat generation — speeds up. Stress can be similarly perceived by the hypothalamus, which may then stimulate steroid secretions from the

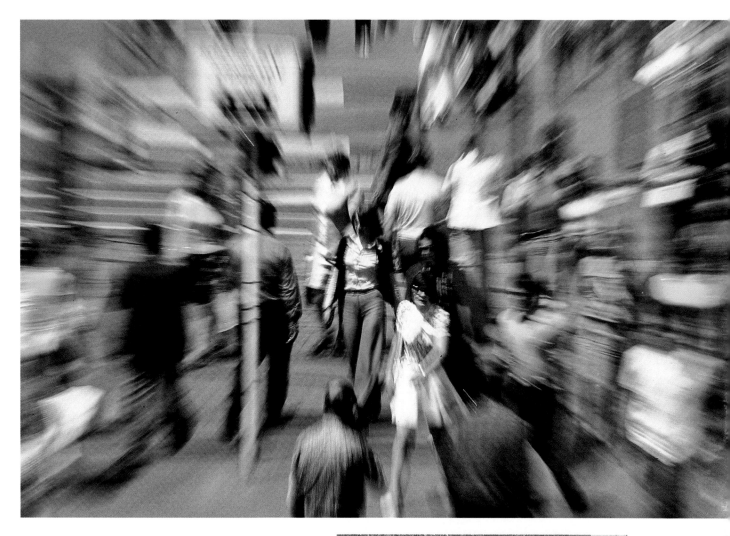

adrenal cortex, although it reduces thyroid activity. The sensing of cold and stress involves the nerves, but it is by means of the neurosecretory cells that changes in hormone secretions can be switched on. This is generally termed the process of "neuro-endocrine integration."

Anterior Pituitary Hormones

Some hormones of the anterior pituitary gland keep up the activity of other endocrine glands — the thyroid, the gonads (ovaries and testes) and the adrenal cortex.

Thyroid-stimulating hormone (TSH) is the pituitary "messenger" which acts on the thyroid gland to stimulate the synthesis and release of the thyroid hormones. It is made up of large protein molecules comprising two subunits (designated α and β), each containing sugar chains. TSH is thus classified as a glycoprotein hormone and is released from the anterior pituitary gland. The hypothalamus stimulates the secretion of TSH through the production of thyrotropin-releasing hormone, and

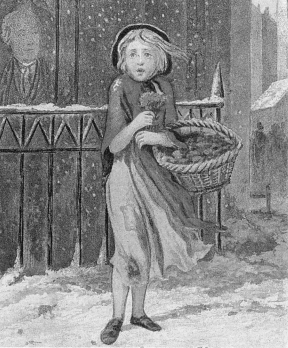

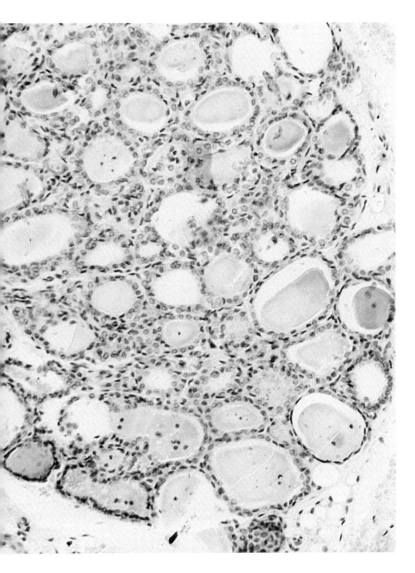

isms by hormones released from target glands are typical in the control of hormone secretions of the anterior pituitary gland, and essential to the overall hormonal balance of the body.

Two trophic hormones produced by the pituitary gland act to maintain gonadal activity: luteinizing hormone (LH) and follicle-stimulating hormone (FSH). The structure of these hormones is similar to TSH in that they are also glycoproteins — in fact the α subunit of the molecule is identical in all three hormones. Evolutionists believe that because of their similarity the three hormones, TSH, LH and FSH evolved from a single ancestral molecule. In many ways this is a reasonable supposition because in lower vertebrates (such as fish), the thyroid hormones are frequently involved in reproductive processes. For example, in sticklebacks thyroxine stimulates a preference for fresh water — these fish migrate from salt water to fresh water in order to spawn.

With the increased demands caused by living on land, it is likely that separate hormones with more specific functions were required and so evolved. Accordingly, two gonadotropic hormones may have evolved rather than a single one, because the gonads have two interrelated functions: firstly to produce gametes (sperm or eggs), and secondly — in common with other endocrine glands — to synthesize and secrete hormones. However, the release of both gonadotropic hormones are controlled by a single hypothalamic releasing factor — luteinizing hormone releasing hormone, otherwise known as gonadotropin-releasing hormone. Like TRH, its secretion rate is regulated both by the feedback effects of gonadal steroids and by influences from the external environment, such as anxiety or desire.

The last anterior pituitary hormone that has a distinct endocrine gland as its target organ is adrenocorticotropic hormone (ACTH), which stimulates the synthesis and secretion of aldosterone, hydrocortisone (cortisol) and corticosterone from the adrenal cortex. ACTH is not a glycoprotein but a simple linear protein made up of a straight chain of thirty-nine amino acids. Its release is stimulated by corticotropin-releasing factor, a hypothalamic hormone whose structure proved difficult to elucidate. However, the hormone was

several factors can alter this rate of production. In animals, cold is a potent stimulator of TRH and hence TSH secretion. Conversely, stress tends to have little or no effect upon the secretion of thyroid-stimulating hormone.

Under normal circumstances the main factor regulating TSH secretion is the circulating levels of the thyroid hormones themselves — triiodothyronine and thyroxine. When their concentrations in the blood increase beyond a certain point, a negative feedback system operates which inhibits the release of TRH, so that there is less stimulation of the thyroid gland by TSH. The release of thyroid hormones into the blood diminishes until the correct levels are reinstated. In converse, when the concentration of thyroid hormones is reduced, the inhibitory effect of the feedback mechanism is decreased: there is an increased release of TSH, and a stimulation of the thyroid glands to produce more thyroid hormones. Such feedback mechan-

Hormones control body rhythms in many different ways. In sticklebacks, for example, the hormone thyroxine plays an important part in the reproductive cycle. The secretion of this hormone at a certain age stimulates their preference for fresh water, causing them to swim from salt to fresh water to spawn. Adrenocorticotropic hormone and hydrocortisone are secreted at a high rate at the end of the night and at a low rate toward the end of the day. These patterns are thought to cause some of the symptoms of jet lag in humans; it takes up to three weeks for the secretions of these hormones to adjust to a new light-dark cycle.

finally broken down in the early 1980s and found to be a peptide of forty-one amino acid constituents. Its secretion is controlled by a negative feedback loop from the circulating concentrations of hydrocortisone and corticosterone.

ACTH is often dubbed the "stress hormone." It is secreted in response to stress and stimulates the release of corticosteroids in the bloodstream. Corticosteroids generally have catabolic effects in the body — they break down proteins to individual amino acids, and stimulate glucose production. They thus increase the concentrations in the blood of energy-providing nutrients, necessary for the response to stress.

The release of ACTH is also closely linked with the light-dark cycle, since the rate of ACTH secretion varies considerably over a twenty-four-hour period. Peak levels of ACTH and hydrocortisone are measured toward the end of the dark period, falling to a nadir in the late hours of the daytime. It is this circadian rhythm of ACTH secretion which is thought to cause some of the symptoms associated with jet lag. If, say, you move from New York to Sydney, across several time zones, for several days your circadian rhythms still operate on the light-dark cycle of New York; your body rhythms are out of phase. In fact it can take up

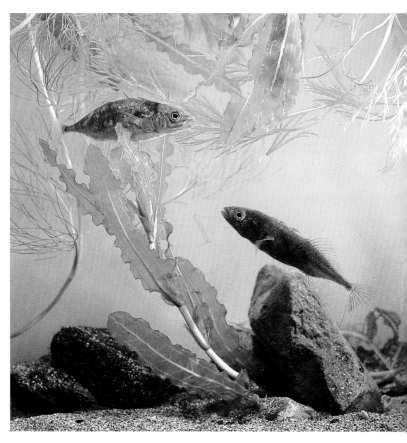

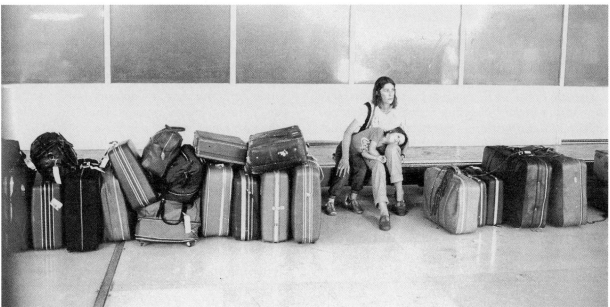

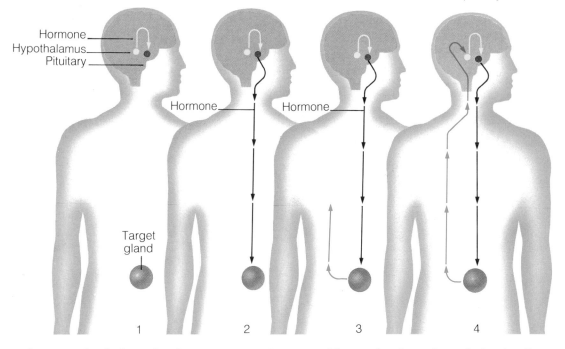

Hormones from the hypothalamus (1) induce the pituitary to secrete hormones (2) which stimulate the target gland to release its hormones (3). These flow to the hypothalamus (4) and inhibit its action.

Bushman women (right) keep their families small partly by breast-feeding their babies for several years. Constant suckling maintains a high level of prolactin in the blood, which reduces fertility.

Hormone
Hypothalamus
Pituitary

Hormone

Hormone

Target gland

1   2   3   4

to three weeks before the hormone secretions synchronize themselves with the new phases of the daily cycle.

The fifth and sixth protein hormones released by the anterior pituitary gland are growth hormone and prolactin (which promotes lactation in nursing mothers); both are similar in structure, and their basic constituents of amino acids (between 190 and 200) are arranged in a spiral fashion. Other similarities between these two hormones are that they do not maintain the activity of a peripheral endocrine gland (unlike TSH, the gonadotropins and ACTH).

Growth hormone (GH) release is stimulated by a growth hormone releasing factor characterized only in 1982. Surprisingly, the material from which this analysis was made did not comprise tons of hypothalamuses purchased from the abattoir, but derived instead from a rare form of pancreatic tumor which autonomously secretes this releasing hormone. Just two patients with such tumors, one from the United States and the other from France, were able to provide enough starting tissue (about six ounces) to extract and analyze the releasing hormone. The second hypothalamic hormone which acts to inhibit the release of growth hormone is called somatostatin.

The predominant hypothalamic effect on prolactin secretion is inhibitory rather than stimulatory, and thus differs from effects connected with other anterior pituitary hormones. The inhibitory factor is dopamine, a relatively small molecule derived from a single amino acid, tyrosine. There is also a prolactin-stimulating factor, but doubt remains as to what it is. The same releasing hormone that stimulates TSH secretion is a likely candidate because it also increases prolactin release; whether TRH is the real physiological stimulator or not is still at this time an open question.

Feedback mechanisms controlling prolactin and growth hormone secretion do exist, but in the form of an "autoregulation" process. The concentrations of the hormones in the blood are monitored by the hypothalamus, which in turn switches on or off the release of the appropriate stimulatory or inhibitory factors. This type of autoregulatory "short" feedback loop replaces the process of feedback by hormones secreted from the target glands of the other anterior pituitary hormones.

Posterior Pituitary Hormones

The second and much smaller lobe of the pituitary gland is the posterior pituitary or neuro-hypophysis. This tiny lobe, a little bigger than a

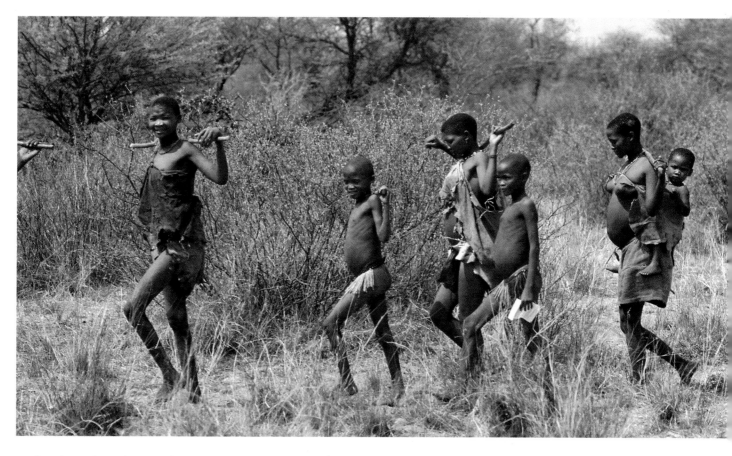

pinhead, and made up almost entirely of nerve endings and blood vessels, releases oxytocin and vasopressin, two peptide hormones which are biochemically very similar to each other. Each is made up of a ring of six amino acids with a "tail" of three amino acids hanging off the circle. Vasopressin release is stimulated when the salt concentration (osmolality) in the blood increases, or when the total volume of the blood in the body decreases. Such changes are detected by "osmo-receptors" in the brain, or volume (stretch) receptors in the major arteries and heart. In this way messages are sent to the neurosecretory cells and they correspondingly pour out more hormone into the circulation. The hormone vasopressin acts on the kidney tubules so that more water is reabsorbed back into the blood and less urine is produced; this is why vasopressin is known also as antidiuretic hormone (ADH). The effect is to help both to dilute the blood salts and to increase the blood volume.

Oxytocin, on the other hand, is involved in milk release in lactating mothers and the contractions of the uterus during labor. (Men also have oxytocin in their pituitaries, but it has no known function.) When babies suck at the breast, sensory receptors in the mother's nipple send neural messages to the hypothalamus, and oxytocin is released. In turn, the oxytocin in the blood stimulates the contraction of the milk ducts in the breast — and milk spurts out of the nipples. The whole process is known as the "milk ejection reflex," and interestingly its operation is particularly susceptible to stress. This is one reason that mothers who are anxious about their ability to breast-feed may have difficulty in releasing their milk when the baby sucks.

Intermediate Pituitary Hormones

The third and smallest lobe of the pituitary gland is the intermediate lobe. Some authorities prefer to ignore this lobe, because in humans there is no distinct intermediate lobe structure (except in the fetus), and its cells are dispersed throughout the posterior or neural lobe. Furthermore, endocrinologists are not even sure of its function, since intermediate lobe tissue is primarily associated with the release of melanocyte-stimulating hormone (α-MSH). This is the hormone that causes skin color changes in lower vertebrates — but no one knows what it does in humans. What has emerged, however, over the last few years is that there are several different types of MSH (designated α, β and γ) and these are all derived from a precursor chemical, which also has ACTH as one of

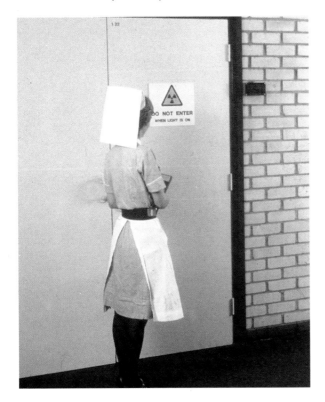

and may also involve an impairment in the hypothalamic control of the gland. Head injuries and radiation may also damage pituitary function; likewise a pituitary hemorrhage after childbirth can cause pituitary necrosis (tissue death) and loss of pituitary secretions.

The history of disorders identified with the pituitary started with the investigation of growth hormone (GH). The hormone, as its name implies, directly promotes growth in soft tissues, cartilage and bone, although its effects on linear growth during childhood involve biochemical intermediaries. These are collectively called somatomedins which, in response to growth hormone, are released from the liver and stimulate the elongation of bones. Children who have a GH deficiency thus show growth failure (dwarfism), and have immature faces and short stature. Hypersecretion of GH conversely produces gigantism, with accelerated growth and an eventual height that may be in excess of eight feet, although body proportions are usually relatively normal.

Gigantism is different from acromegaly, which describes the characteristics of a GH excess that occurs in adults when linear growth has stopped. Enlarged hands and feet, coarse facial features and an elongated face are typical of acromegaly. Various metabolic disturbances — notably diabetes mellitus — are also linked with excessive GH secretions.

Deficiency or excess may also occur in the secretion of prolactin, the milk hormone. In pregnancy the mother's prolactin-secreting pituitary cells enlarge, and so does the pituitary gland itself. Prolactin secretion rises steadily over the nine-month period, and when the baby is born and the placenta stops producing steroids, prolactin is free to stimulate milk production. Suckling maintains a relatively high output of this hormone, and thus lactation can continue for long periods after childbirth.

The only known clinical effect of deficient prolactin secretion is the inability to lactate shortly after childbirth. Hypersecretion in a non-pregnant woman can conversely cause inappropriate lactation (galactorrhea), in which the breasts are engorged with milk and can be extremely painful. High prolactin levels may also cause infertility and

its constituents. From this same precursor the whole family of opioid peptides in the brain and pituitary are formed, about which there is more at the end of the chapter.

Pituitary Gland Disorders

The constant and efficient activities of the pituitary gland, pouring chemical messages into the bloodstream, are evidently extremely important. But what happens when things go wrong? The best way of answering the question is to look at why the pituitary goes wrong at all.

The most common cause of pituitary malfunction is a benign tumor of the anterior lobe of the pituitary (adenoma). The tumor cells themselves may secrete specific hormones and so produce a disorder reflecting the excess of one or more of the pituitary hormones (hyperpituitarism). In addition, the enlargement of the pituitary gland resulting from the tumor can cause pressure and thus damage the gland itself; in more severe cases, such damage can extend up into the hypothalamus. This causes reduction of pituitary secretions (hypopituitarism),

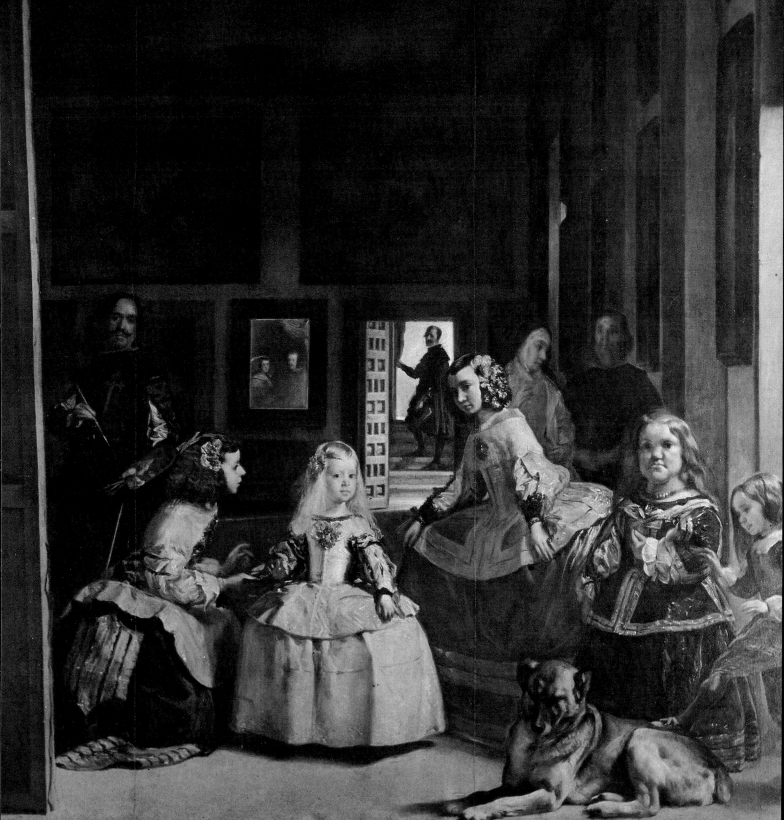

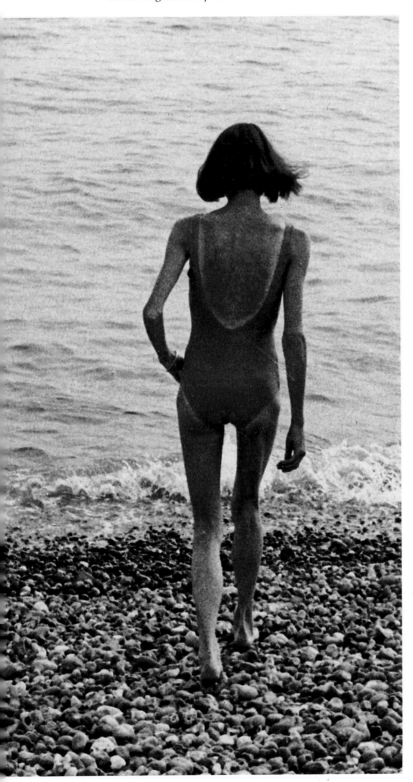

inhibit menstruation — an effect which may account for up to fifteen per cent of infertility in women. It is certainly the cause of reduced fertility after childbirth, and this is why lactation has been termed "nature's contraceptive" — a natural way to space out subsequent conceptions. However, lactation and high prolactin secretions do not guarantee infertility, as many mothers can testify, and so contraception is always recommended after childbirth, irrespective of the choice to breast-feed or to bottle-feed. In men, an excess of prolactin may lower levels of gonadotropins and testosterone, causing impotence and infertility.

Excesses or deficiencies in the gonadotropins affect sexuality. Sexual precocity (early sexual development) results when excess gonadotropins are released in young children; a deficiency on the other hand delays or prevents the development of sexual characteristics. If a deficiency occurs in an adult, secondary sex characteristics begin to atrophy; there is a loss of pubic hair, of fertility and of libido. Probably the most common cause of a gonadotropin deficiency is found in young girls whose menstruation ceases because of stress or weight loss; its severest form is encountered in anorexia nervosa.

In many patients suffering from Cushing's syndrome, excess production of hormones from the adrenal cortex, the cause is a hypersecretion of ACTH from the pituitary gland. There is therefore an overstimulation of the adrenal cortex and an excessive production of hydrocortisone and corticosterone. It is, however, a rare disease, and primarily affects women in the age-group thirty to fifty years. The adrenal steroids have a generalized catabolic effect on the body's metabolism, and when they are secreted to excess there is muscle weakness in the arms and legs, and a decreased density of bone (especially in the spine), which predisposes to fractures and bone pain. The skin becomes thin and bruises easily, and increased fat is laid down over the trunk of the body because the steroids stimulate fat deposition. Androgens, also produced by the adrenal cortex, cause masculinization and infertility.

A loss of adrenal gland secretions results in Addison's disease, but this is very rarely caused by an insufficiency of ACTH secretion: it normally

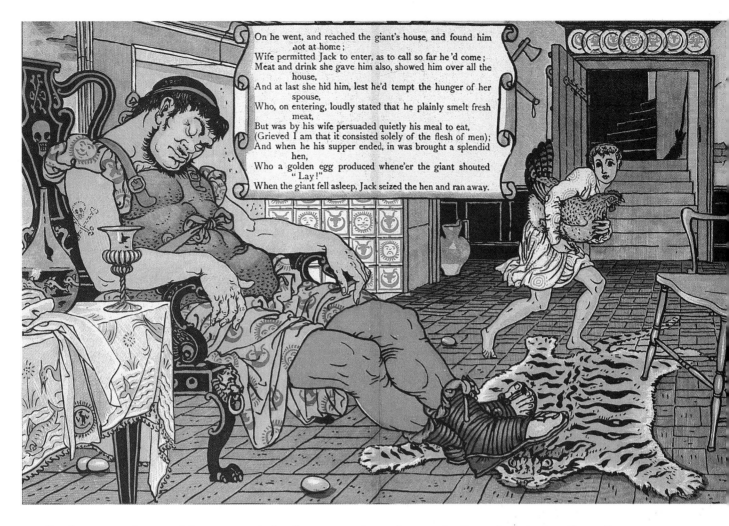

On he went, and reached the giant's house, and found him
   not at home;
Wife permitted Jack to enter, as to call so far he'd come;
Meat and drink she gave him also, showed him over all the
   house,
And at last she hid him, lest he'd tempt the hunger of her
   spouse,
Who, on entering, loudly stated that he plainly smelt fresh
   meat,
But was by his wife persuaded quietly his meal to eat,
(Grieved I am that it consisted solely of the flesh of men);
And when he his supper ended, in was brought a splendid
   hen,
Who a golden egg produced whene'er the giant shouted
   "Lay!"
When the giant fell asleep, Jack seized the hen and ran away.

results from a primary defect present in the adrenal gland itself.

The last of the hormones of the anterior pituitary gland is thyroid-stimulating hormone. The main cause of overstimulation of the thyroid gland is Graves' disease, but this not the result of excessive TSH secretion. In fact, inappropriate secretion of TSH rarely occurs. A deficiency of TSH release produces, of course, symptoms of hypothyroidism, accompanied by the tiredness and lethargy typical of the condition.

No cases have been reported in which a tumor of the posterior pituitary gland has produced an excess of either oxytocin or antidiuretic hormone (vasopressin), although an excessive secretion of antidiuretic hormone can occur as a result of a wide variety of clinical conditions. Such "inappropriate" secretion of vasopressin leads to a low sodium concentration in the blood and the production of highly concentrated urine. In contrast, a deficiency of the hormone, a condition called diabetes insipidus, usually resulting from a head injury or brain surgery, causes an insatiable thirst and massive urine production of up to ten times the normal daily volume.

The manifestations of a diseased or injured pituitary gland amply illustrate its importance. Although the effects of individual hormone excesses or deficiencies have been described, frequently the secretion of more than one of the pituitary hormones is affected. This is particularly true in cases of hormone deficiency — which rarely occurs in isolation.

What is Neuroendocrinology?

The discovery of hypothalamic nerve cells that released hormones into the circulation, rather than releasing neurotransmitters into the synaptic cleft, gave rise to a now burgeoning field of research: neuroendocrinology. At first this field seemed clearly defined — it concerned the way in which the hypothalamus controls pituitary secretions, and the interactions between the hormones and the relevant nerves.

Then scientists began to find that what had been called "hypothalamic hormones" were not strictly

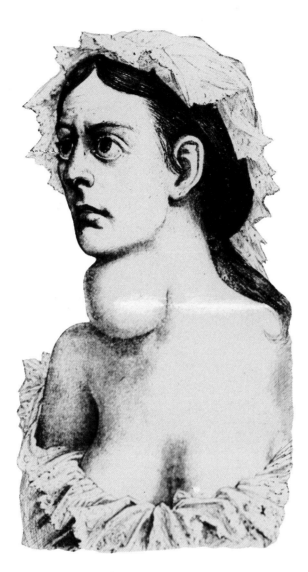

An enlarged thyroid gland (the bulge on the woman's throat) and protruding eyeballs are symptomatic of Graves' disease, also known as exophthalmic goiter. This condition results from the overactivity of the gland, leading to the toxic condition thyrotoxicosis. It occurs more frequently among females than males.

hypothalamic in origin. They were discovered in other parts of the brain and in the spinal cord, then found even outside of the central nervous system. The growth hormone inhibiting hormone, somatostatin, serves as a good example. Much of it is found in the pancreas, where it inhibits insulin and glucagon release; it is also in the spinal cord, the sympathetic ganglia, the retina of the eye, and throughout the brain. Similarly, thyrotropin-releasing hormone is found in many parts of the nervous system, and in other tissues including the eye, gut and placenta.

In fact, all of the classic "hypothalamic hormones" can be found in other areas of the brain — and, to complicate the picture even further, both the hypothalamus and pituitary gland are stuffed full of other peptides which are not known to be released as hormones. So where does neuroendocrinology begin and end, and what marks the differentiation between a neurohormone and a neurotransmitter?

One family of peptides which does perhaps appear to be intimately related with neuroendocrine integration are the opioidlike peptides — so named because some of them have actions similar to those of the opiate drugs, morphine and heroin; β-endorphin, ACTH, the melanocyte-stimulating hormones and enkephalins are some of the many members of this family. There are large amounts of opioid peptides in the hypothalamus and pituitary gland. Generally they seem to act as modulators in the control of other hormone secretion, but they may be particularly important as mediators in the feedback mechanisms which operate to maintain stable hormone secretions. They may also play a part in relating changes in the environment, such as the light-dark cycle, temperature or stressful situations, to changes in hormone secretions. The answer is that nobody really knows the answer — or indeed if these apparent functions comprise the whole story.

So there are still many questions concerning the neuroendocrine system. To unravel the complex machinery by which hormone feedback mechanisms and neural inputs from our environment are integrated in the hypothalamus and then translated into an endocrine signal from the neurosecretory (transducer) cells will prove an awesome task.

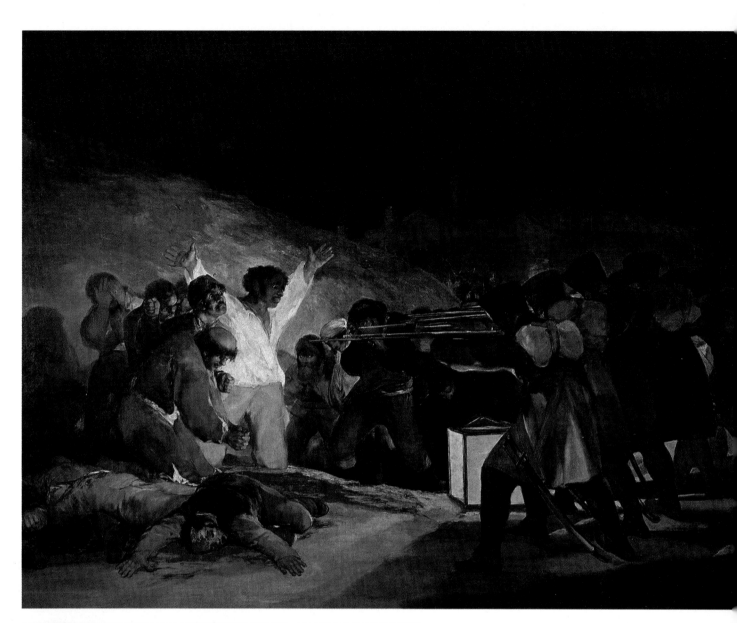

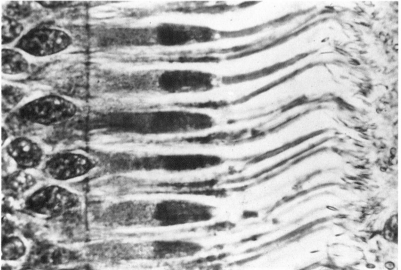

The hormones, such as epinephrine, that are released in stressful conditions (above), result in behavior patterns such as staring eyes, rigidity and breathlessness. These hormones, it is thought, may be regulated by opioid peptides which are found in the pituitary. Hormones are secreted not only by the endocrine glands but have also been found to be released from nerve cells in the retina (left). The study of the interrelation of hormones and nerves and of peptides and hormones is called neuroendocrinology.

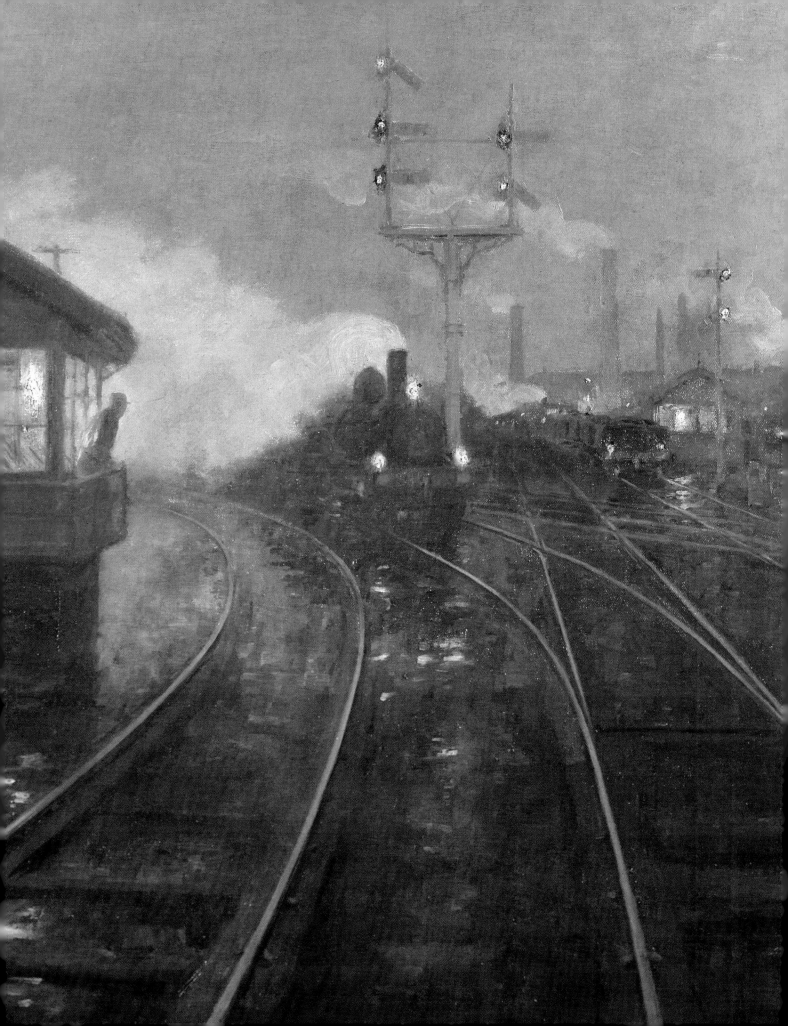

Chapter 4

Hormonal Harmony

In Roman mythology Mercury was the messenger of the Gods. The human body has its own version of Mercury: the chemical messengers known as hormones. But whereas the Gods had only one messenger, the body has many hormones which comprise its complex chemical communications network. Just as Mercury, who merely acted as a messenger and was not directly involved in the business of the Gods, so hormones carry chemical information from various glands to tissues which then act on the instructions.

Without hormones the body would be like a large and complex army without any battle commands and therefore no chance of winning a war. Hormones trigger responses from target cells, either locally or far from their point of origin in an endocrine gland. They are transported around the body in the bloodstream. Their overall responsibility is to maintain the metabolic equilibrium of the body by compensating, through messages, for disruptive changes — that is, they maintain the status quo. The way hormones do this involves a series of reactions, starting with their synthesis in endocrine glands and ending with feedback mechanisms which control their release. The process can be likened to the action of a thermostat, which "senses" the temperature in a room, say, and turns the heat on when the room becomes too cold or turns it off when the room conversely becomes too warm.

Depending on their biochemical structure and the manner in which they communicate their messages, hormones can be categorized into one of the following three groups: protein and polypeptide hormones, steroid hormones and miscellaneous hormones; all are synthesized from various chemical building blocks in the cytoplasm of cells. Protein and polypeptide hormones, synthesized from amino acids, are the most common. Steroid hormones are derived from cholesterol. Miscellaneous hormones, which do

The switches on a railroad track dictate the direction in which the train carrying its cargo will travel. In the same way, endocrine organs release hormones that have specific targets in the body.

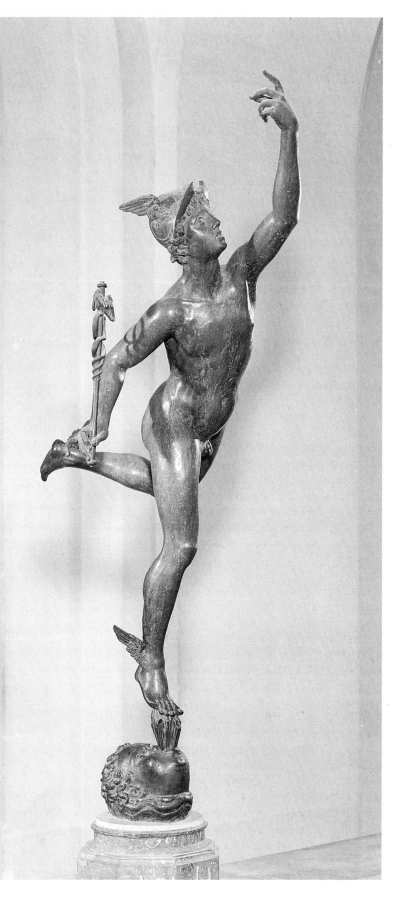

not quite fit into either of the other two groups, include locally-acting hormones which take effect upon cells and tissues in the actual environment in which the hormones are first put together. Called autocoids, these hormones include acetylcholine, the neurotransmitter.

Hormone synthesis

The biochemical factory which produces protein and polypeptide hormones has its "generating plant" in the nucleus of an endocrine cell. The blueprints produced there are exported out of the nucleus and used to direct the assembly of components at cytoplasmic structures in the cell called ribosomes. The initial process at the "generating plant," in which RNA is manufactured at the chromosomes with DNA acting as a template, is called transcription. The assembly stage, in which RNA controls the formation of protein and polypeptide molecules at the ribosomes, is known as translation. Once synthesized, the hormone molecule migrates toward a cellular organelle known as the Golgi apparatus (so named in 1898 for its discoverer, the Italian pathologist Camillo Golgi), where it is packaged within a membrane-bound vesicle.

Steroid hormones are made to order, much as burgers in a fast-food restaurant. When an endocrine cell receives an order, for instance in the form of a nervous stimulus, an enzyme (or enzymes) is activated. This induces a series of reactions whereby the building blocks stored in the cytoplasm are put together to form the finished steroid molecules. Like asking the checkout staff for a burger with everything on it, the message goes to the cooks telling them what to prepare, and back comes a burger with lettuce, tomato, relish, mustard and whatever other side orders are required. The miscellaneous hormones also fit into this "fast-food" category.

Sometimes, hormones are produced directly from inactive precursor molecules called prohormones, which are usually proteins or polypeptides. For example, insulin is formed from the cleavage of a molecule known as proinsulin; the splitting occurs in storage granules in the cytoplasm of the islet cells of the pancreas. Proinsulin has no other use than to provide insulin when it splits; the

Organized strategies which rely on the relaying of information to and from the control center for their success are just as essential for a battle (below) as for endocrine glands. The pancreas is a command center which monitors the blood glucose level. When the level is high it sends out insulin from its islets of Langerhans (bottom), which increases the passage of glucose into cells, restoring the normal level.

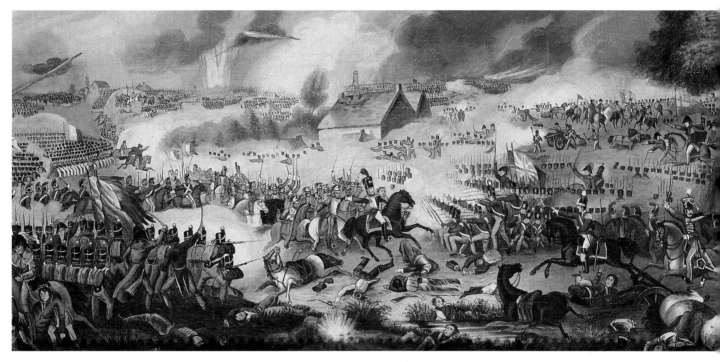

process is therefore rather like cutting a key from a piece of otherwise unusable metal.

Storage and Release

An advantage of these inactive prohormones is that they can be stored in the cytoplasm in a form that can be converted quickly when needed. The storage of inactive molecules or proteins and polypeptides in the cytoplasmic granules of endocrine cells is necessary to protect them from being broken down by cell enzymes. It also prevents hormones from acting upon the cells which make them. But with the made-to-order steroid hormones storage is not necessary because they are released into the bloodstream as soon as they are manufactured.

The release of protein and polypeptide hormones into the blood from their imprisonment within secretory granules follows the stimulation of their respective endocrine cells. The hormones are expelled by "exocytosis," in which the granule fuses with the cellular membrane and by a complex mechanism throws out its contents into the bloodstream. This dramatic process of secretion is, in many respects, similar to the release of

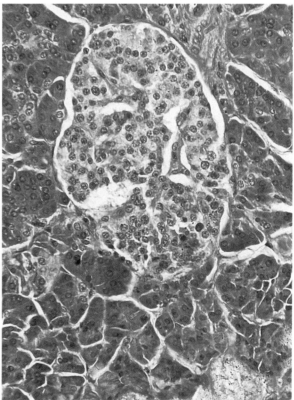

Feedback mechanisms are negative or positive. Negative feedback (below) operates when a person eats a meal and glucose is absorbed, raising the blood glucose level. Insulin is secreted from the pancreas, which metabolizes the glucose and stabilizes the blood glucose level. Positive feedback is exemplified in a woman about to give birth (bottom). Oxytocin is secreted before labor but, when the baby's head reaches the birth canal, messages are sent to the hypothalamus. It stimulates the pituitary to release more oxytocin, which causes the contractions that push the baby out. Once the baby has been born, oxytocin release stops.

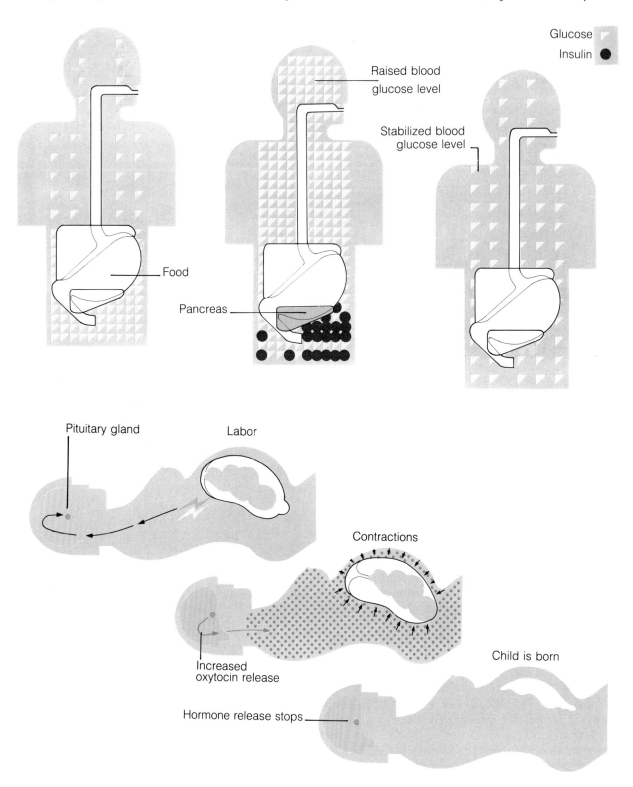

Glucose

Insulin

Raised blood glucose level

Stabilized blood glucose level

Food

Pancreas

Pituitary gland

Labor

Contractions

Increased oxytocin release

Child is born

Hormone release stops

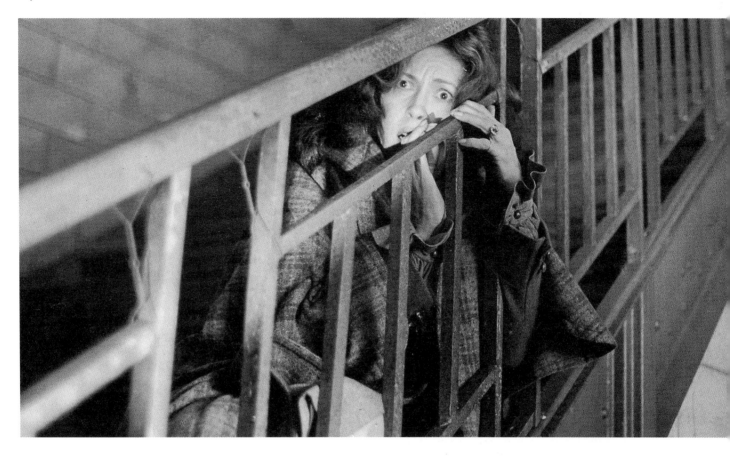

The Eyes of Laura Mars is a vivid depiction of the reactions of a person who sees something alarming. Epinephrine is released in these situations, alerting the body to respond to the crisis.

neurotransmitters from nerve endings — both processes need the presence of calcium ions which, in endocrine cells are necessary for exocytosis to take place. The release of steroids is not as violent as exocytosis. Once synthesized, these lipid-soluble molecules can immediately and easily pass through the cell membrane into the bloodstream. The miscellaneous hormones are secreted by either route, exocytosis or straight diffusion.

Transport and Excretion

Most people have a bank account and also carry some cash. The money in the bank is stored there for safe keeping and can be called on by using a check when needed, whereas cash is for immediate use. The human body's system for moving hormones around can be thought of in a similar way. Freely circulating protein and polypeptide hormones are like cash — they are transported around the body in the bloodstream, whereas other steroid and thyroid hormones are either free (active) or protein-bound and inactive. The binding protects these hormones from inactivation by other substances in the blood and keeps them in a stored (but circulating) form as a reservoir from which they are released and become active when their target cells need them. It is as if the target cells write out a check and the bank of protein-bound hormones thereupon cashes that check in the form of unbound hormones.

Sometimes we need to change our currency from dollars to, say, pounds. In the body some hormones undergo a similar change of "currency" when they are secreted in one active form and then chemically modified in another part of the body to become a different hormone with new functions. The "banks" in which these changes take place include the liver, brain, breast and adipose tissue. For example the hormone estrogen (secreted by the ovary) undergoes the process of peripheral conver-

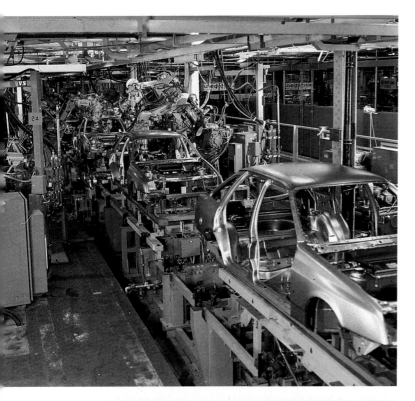

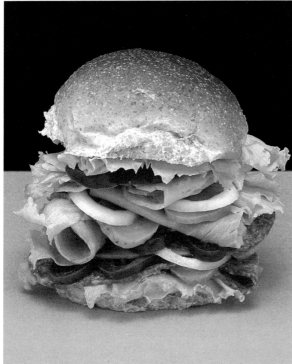

sion, by tissues far from the original endocrine gland, into testosterone, which has a different action from its original one.

Once a hormone has been "spent," it is excreted in the urine. Efficient excretion is as important to the body as is good ventilation to a house. When the body has reaped the benefit of a hormone's effect on its target cells, the hormone is usually inactivated or broken down by its target tissue or, more commonly, by the liver, which combines it with other substances to form a water-soluble substance. This can then be secreted into the bile and excreted in the feces, or can enter the bloodstream to be excreted by the kidneys. The kidneys themselves sometimes inactivate hormones and excrete them into the urine.

How Hormones Work

There are still gaps in present-day knowledge about how hormones exert their effects on target cells, because the human body is such a vastly complex biochemical maze. It is known, however, that individual hormones recognize their specific target cells, and this recognition depends on the presence of hormone-specific cell receptors.

The hormone acts like a key and the cell receptor like a lock which only one key will open. Sometimes, different hormones have the same actions, analagous to using a slightly different key which, with a little bit of forcing, will also open the lock. For example, oxytocin (which helps the womb contract during childbirth) and the hormone vasopressin (which has antidiuretic properties) have similar structures and actions. Vasopressin can cause stimulation of the womb under certain conditions and oxytocin has some antidiuretic uses in administration.

There are two main sites of hormone recognition: the plasma membrane around the cell, and the cytoplasmic receptors within the cell itself. Protein and polypeptide hormones are usually unable to penetrate the cell membrane and therefore need to bind to membrane receptors. Hormones that are fat-soluble, such as the steroids, can pass through the plasma membranes of their target cells by diffusion and attach to cytoplasmic receptors contained inside the cell.

The ways in which hormones exert their effects at

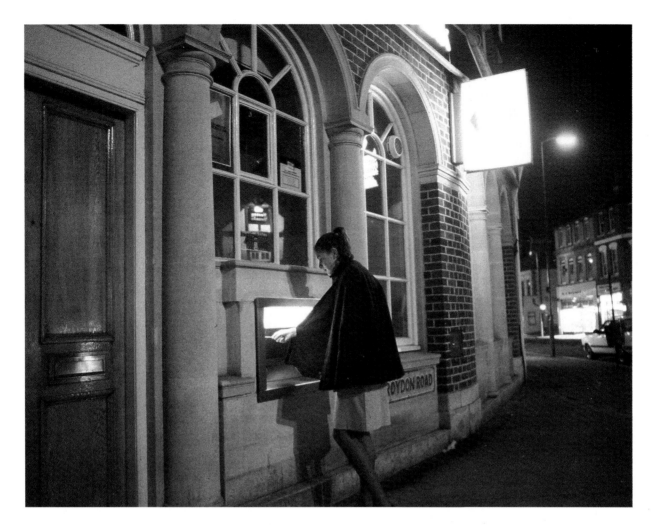

receptors are thought to be three. Firstly, there is the mechanism in which a hormone has a direct effect on the plasma membrane of its target cell, altering the transport of ions or molecules through it. The second way may involve binding to membrane receptors which, in turn, activates cytoplasmic systems to produce "second messengers." These initiate a series of processes, each characteristic of the particular hormone, which either influence an intracellular enzyme system or signal the production of more protein.

There are several possible "second messengers" which scientists believe exist within the cell, including prostaglandins, calcium ions and cyclic adenosine 3':5'-monophosphate (cyclic AMP), which has attracted the most interest. Cyclic AMP is a product of adenosine triphosphate (ATP), the body's energy-carrying chemical vehicle. It seems that the production of cyclic AMP activates enzymes (called protein kinases) within the cytoplasm. These enzymes then set off a chain of intracellular events.

The first hint that one of ATP's breakdown products could have such an important role came in 1958, a year in which experiments showed that the formation of cyclic AMP was a vital step in the liver's conversion of glycogen to glucose, and that it was the hormone epinephrine which sparked off the release of cyclic AMP. The action of the thyrotropin-releasing hormone and the gonadotropin-releasing hormone on the anterior pituitary (adenohypophysis), as well as the effects of epinephrine and glucagon on the liver and adipose tissue, and the effects of vasopressin on the kidney, are all systems also thought to involve cyclic AMP as a second messenger. It may also be possible that cyclic AMP influences a "third messenger," which then activates a string of intracellular activities.

The third mode of hormone action involves those hormones, such as steroids, which are capable of slipping through the plasma membrane and combining with cytoplasmic receptors. The combined hormone and receptor change into an active form and move into the nucleus. It seems that these hormone-receptor complexes are able to influence

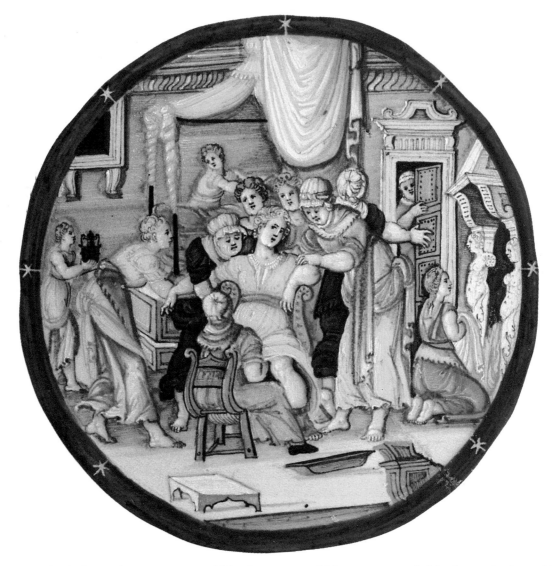

protein synthesis by acting on genes within the nucleus. One exciting theory about how this works involves the combination of the hormone-receptor complexes with a regulator gene, which is effectively a general in charge of adjacent genes. These genes can be thought of as the general's troops whose job it is to enforce the synthesis of protein (by synthesis of RNA from the DNA in the chromosomes, causing amino acids to be linked together to form proteins).

Normally, the general stops or represses the activity of the troops, but if the hormone-receptor complex distracts the general's attention, by attachment to the gene site, then the troops could get on with the protein synthesis and thus exert a detectable hormonal response. This theory is known as the gene de-repression theory because the hormone-receptor complex inhibits the influence of the regulator gene. However, the more recent direct gene-activation theory proposes that

steroid hormones probably do not bother with the general but instruct the troops directly themselves, thus instigating protein synthesis. Both explanations may in fact be accurate.

Endocrine control

The glands that secrete hormones are like command centers which need constant information on the performance of their troops. In the human body there are many feedback mechanisms which provide such information and instruct each gland on the amount of hormone to be released. Feedback can be either negative or positive. In negative feedback the rate of release of a hormone from an endocrine gland is regulated by the blood concentration of the chemical it controls (such as blood glucose in the case of glucagon secretion), or by the blood level of the hormone itself. When the blood level of such a chemical gets too high or too low, the endocrine gland reacts by secreting either less or more hormone — so much as to bring the level back to normal.

An important example of regulation occurs when the concentration of glucose in the blood rises, for instance after eating a meal. The endocrine cells in the islets of Langerhans in the pancreas detect the increase of blood glucose and respond by increasing the rate of insulin secretion, which then affects its target cells to bring the glucose level back down to normal. Insulin controls the movement of glucose into the liver and its secretion back into the bloodstream when energy is needed.

An example of negative feedback, which is less direct, involves the relationship between blood glucose concentration and the release of the growth hormone somatotropin from the front part of the pituitary gland (the anterior pituitary or adenohypophysis). A lower level of glucose concentration in the blood influences the inhibition by the brain of somatostatin (the hypothalamic inhibitory hormone) and the secretion of somatotropin-releasing factor (SRF), which together control the release of somatotropin from the anterior pituitary. The presence of somatotropin inhibits the action of insulin, which raises the level of glucose in the blood, which in turn results in greater secretion of somatostatin and a reduction in the release of SRF, thereby reducing the secretion of somatotropin. Several other adenohypophysial hormones, including corticotropin and thyrotropin, are similarly under the control of releasing and inhibitory factors which operate a negative feedback system.

Positive feedback is the opposite of negative feedback. A hormone acts as a stimulus, either directly or indirectly, for its own production — which must obviously be short-lived or self-limiting to prevent an infinite increase in hormone levels. A good example of indirect positive feedback occurs when the hormone oxytocin acts on a woman's womb to increase contractions during childbirth. As the baby begins to pass through the birth canal, the ensuing pressure triggers nerve impulses to the brain, where they stimulate oxytocin secretion from the posterior pituitary and thus stimulate further contractions of the womb. It is as if the womb is telling the brain: "Send more oxytocin, otherwise the baby won't be

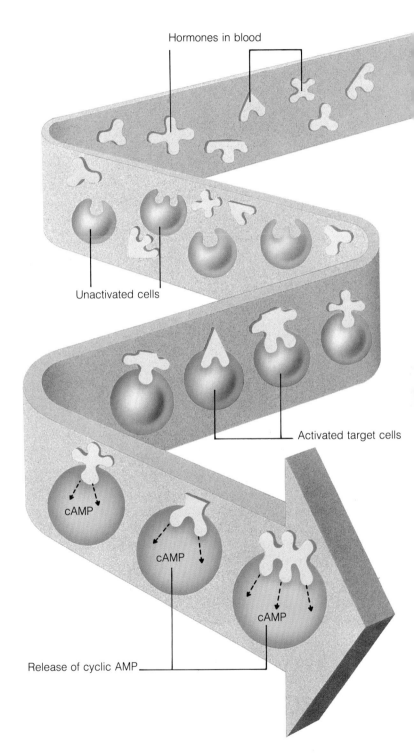

Hormones in blood

Unactivated cells

Activated target cells

cAMP

cAMP

cAMP

Release of cyclic AMP

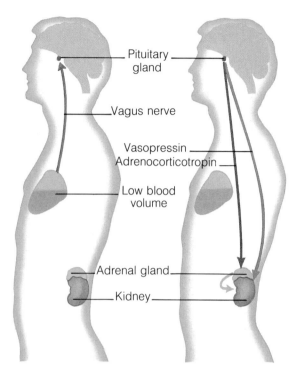

The myths and legends that have grown up around giants such as Goya's Colossus were probably based on gigantic figures from real life whose size resulted from an excess of growth hormone during their youth.

Hormones play an important part in the regulation of blood volume. When fluid passes from the circulation system into tissues, the blood volume decreases. This condition is communicated by the vagus nerve to the pituitary, which secretes the hormones vasopressin and adrenocorticotropin. The first hormone goes to the kidneys to reduce their excretion of fluid, and the second goes to the adrenal glands. These glands send aldosterone to the kidneys and induces them to retain salt. In this way the blood volume is increased.

able to get out." Once the baby is born, the nerve impulses to the brain cease and oxytocin release also stops.

Another form of endocrine control, particularly useful when the human body is in danger, involves the nervous system. For example, epinephrine (adrenaline) is released following nervous stimulation of the innermost part (medulla) of the adrenal glands, sometimes as a consequence of the brain's perception of a situation which poses a threat or is frightening. As a result, the body becomes alert and ready to deal with an impending crisis. In addition, the blood-pressure-regulating juxtaglomerular cells of the kidney, the insulin-producing beta cells of the islets of Langerhans in the pancreas, and the pituitary gland are also stimulated when the body is in danger, initially signaled into action through the nervous system.

Hormones and Growth

The growth of the human body from conception to adult size is remarkable in that a fully grown human is thousands of times larger than the fertilized ovum from which he or she originated. Growth on such a scale requires the assistance of hormones, the most abundant of which is somatotropin, the growth hormone, produced by the pituitary gland. This hormone has a dramatic effect on body development, promoting the growth of soft tissues, cartilage and bone. It exerts its vital effect on the transport of amino acids through cell membranes and by influencing the liver to synthesize a group of polypeptides known as somatomedins, which also help stimulate growth.

But just like machines — even new ones — the body does not always perform perfectly, and sometimes the pituitary gland secretes too much or too little of the growth hormone. An excess can in extreme cases lead to gigantism. The most severe recorded example of this condition is an American man who in the 1940s reached a height of 8 feet 11 inches. At the other end of the scale, where there is an extreme deficiency of the hormone, the Tom Thumb or circus-freak kind of dwarf is the result. Typically, a "pituitary" dwarf is not much more than two feet tall, but mercifully such people have normal intelligence and their bodies have normal proportions despite small dimensions.

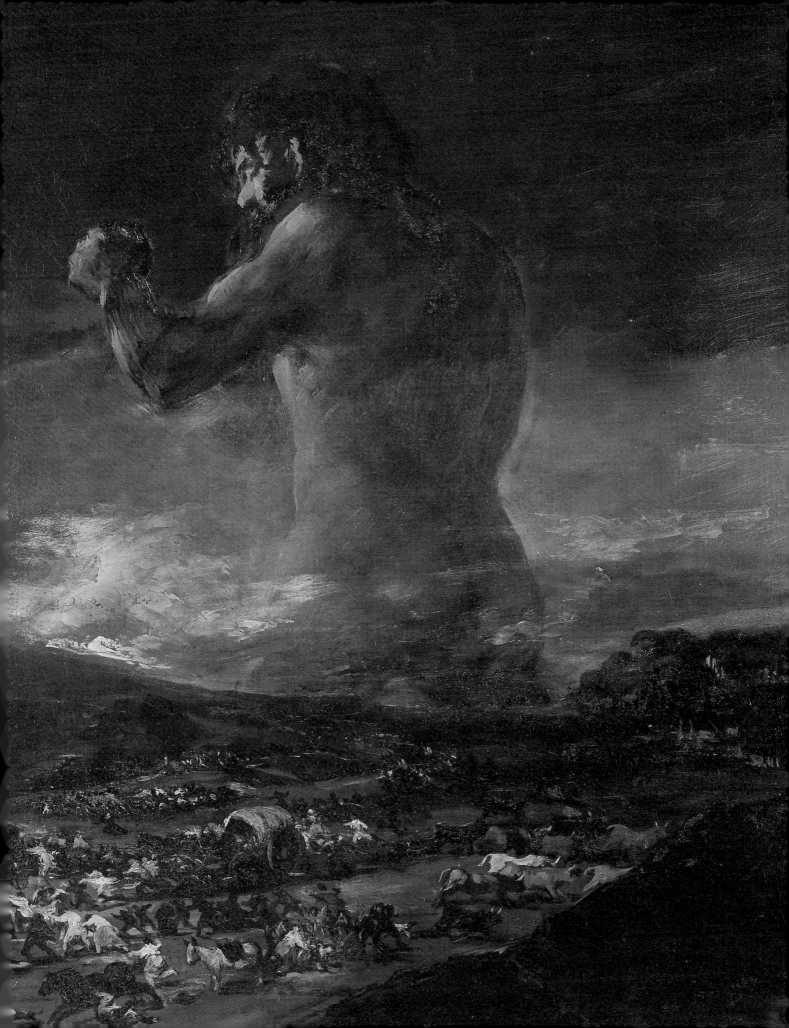

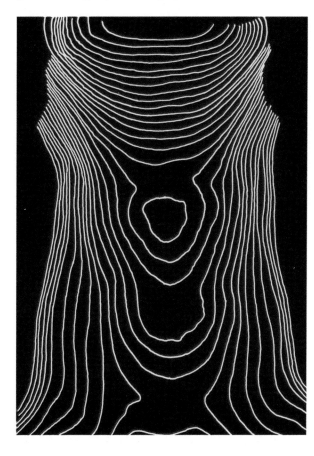 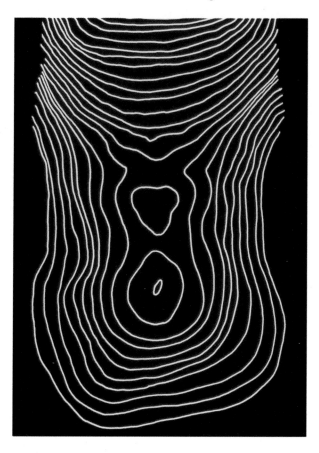

The body is also indebted to the thyroid gland for its role in normal development. The gland's two chief hormones are thyroxine (also known as T_4) and triiodothyronine (T_3). Both regulate the metabolic rate of the body and increase protein synthesis. A deficiency of thyroid hormones leads to an almost complete cessation of skeletal growth, and can result in cretinism (severely retarded physical and mental development) in a child or myxedema in an adult.

Insulin, as well as being of vital importance in the control of blood sugar levels (deficiency of this hormone can lead to the debilitating condition diabetes mellitus), is also important in growth, because insulin directly stimulates protein synthesis without which growth cannot occur. This is dramatically illustrated by the stunted growth of diabetic infants with insulin deficiency, in comparison with oversized babies born to diabetic mothers. (In the latter case, the mother's insulin treatment leads to correspondingly high insulin levels in the fetus growing within her.)

Local hormones

As well as hormones carried in the bloodstream from their glandular origins to their target organs, there is a group of hormones which act on tissues or cells in the immediate neighborhood of their site of formation. These local hormones, called autocoids, have between them an enormous range of functions and play significant roles in health and disease. They include catecholamines, acetylcholine, histamine, kinin peptides and prostaglandins, as detailed below.

The catecholamines, which include dopamine (a precursor of norepinephrine), norepinephrine and epinephrine, are produced by the adrenal medulla and by certain nerve endings. Their functions include increasing the heart's rate and force of contraction to supply oxygen-carrying blood rapid-

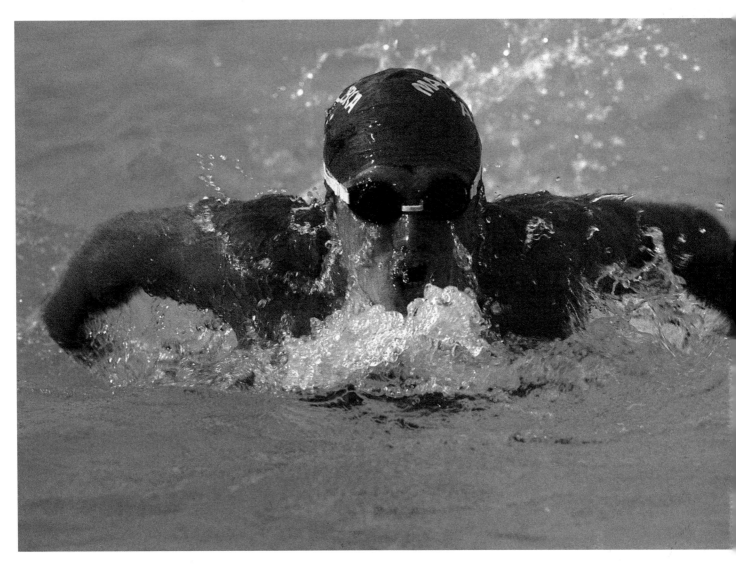

ly to muscles, such as those of an athlete in need of extra oxygen. They also help increase or decrease the amount of air the lungs can breathe by regulating the dilatation of bronchial and bronchiolar muscles.

Catecholamines are also important in helping the body digest and absorb nutrients from food passing through the gastrointestinal tract. They do this by controlling the secretion of gut enzymes, by controlling peristalsis (the process whereby food is squeezed along the tract), and by stimulating contraction of intestinal sphincters which prevent food from moving through the gut. And as when the body experiences fear, catecholamine release appears to cause symptoms of anxiety, such as blanching, sweating, loss of bladder control, increased breathing and shaky hands. These effects are caused primarily by an increase in epinephrine.

Another fascinating autocoid with an interesting historical background is acetylcholine. It was first discovered, in 1867, by the German chemist Adolf von Baeyer. But because the medical men of his time were suspicious of chemists, von Baeyer was prevented from carrying out pioneering research by their refusal to grant him a position in the medical faculty where he would have had better access to human tissue for experimentation. It is ironic that today both professions depend on each other to produce a sophisticated arsenal of drugs that are the basis of modern medical practice.

Following this unfortunate beginning, interest in acetylcholine did not revive until after 1900. It was a student called T. R. Elliot at Cambridge University, England, who in 1905 discovered that an epinephrine-like substance was released by nerves in immediate contact with effector tissues. The substance was acetylcholine, and since his remarkable discovery it has been established that acetylcholine is vital in the transmission of impulses along parasympathetic nerves which

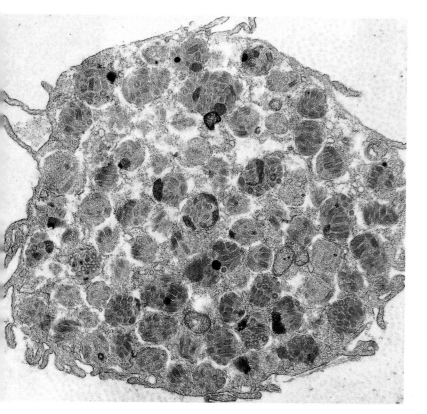

An electron micrograph of a human mast cell reveals granules which contain histamine, an autocoid that is involved in the inflammation symptomatic of many allergies, such as hay fever.

stimulate digestion (where it initiates hormone release), bladder movement, bowel emptying, sexual function, dilatation of the iris of the eye, salivary gland secretion and sweating — an impressive catalog for the actions of a single chemical!

An autocoid which can be a friend or foe to the body is histamine. On the plus side it enlarges blood vessels and thus increases blood supply to the tissues. But on the minus side abnormally large quantities of histamine produce an allergic reaction. Increased histamine production occurs in response to the presence of a particular antigen, such as pollen, dust or even certain foods, and leads to swelling and reddening of the skin. A wound or some cases of shock elicits a similar response. In rare cases of extreme allergy, in which the symptoms are spread throughout the body — a condition known as anaphylaxis — the reaction is so severe that heart failure, circulatory collapse and even death can occur.

Autocoids which have recently generated great interest in the scientific world are the peptides known as endorphins and enkephalins. These opioidlike substances are present in the brain and thought to have important roles in human behavior and in the perception of pain. As research reveals more about exactly what chemical messages these peptides deliver, an era of better treatment of pain may arrive and more help may become available for people with certain emotional and personality disorders.

The most exciting of all the autocoids, whose discovery also represents one of the greatest advances in medicine in this century, are a remarkable group of substances known as prostaglandins. They were first identified almost simultaneously in the early 1930s by two different teams of scientists, Kurzrok and Lieb, and Goldblatt and von Euler. These workers observed that an extract of human semen could cause contractions of isolated intestinal and uterine smooth muscle. They could not have realized at the time that the substances they had discovered would turn out to have the most varied actions of any naturally occurring compound.

It was von Euler who isolated the active compounds in semen and discovered that they were fatty acids, and named them prostaglandins. The name originated from the mistaken belief that they were secreted by the prostate gland; it is now known that they come from the seminal vesicles in the testes.

Unfortunately, the great significance of the prostaglandin discovery was lost to the medical profession until the 1960s, when interest was resurrected. The Swedish scientists Bergström and Sjövall isolated and identified two classes of prostaglandin in sheep seminal vesicles and called them prostaglandin E (PGE), which was soluble in ether, and prostaglandin F (PGF), which was soluble in phosphate buffer (in Swedish phosphate is spelled with an F, hence PGF). Yet another class of prostaglandins, PGA, was discovered in rabbit kidney medulla in 1963.

Since the 1960s there has been a boom in research into prostaglandins as their importance has been recognized, and other types have been discovered. These hormones have a physiological effect far from their point of release and are regarded as local

Vitamin K crystals (below) are an important agent in blood coagulation. Prostaglandins work against vitamin K by preventing platelets from clumping and forming a blood clot (bottom).

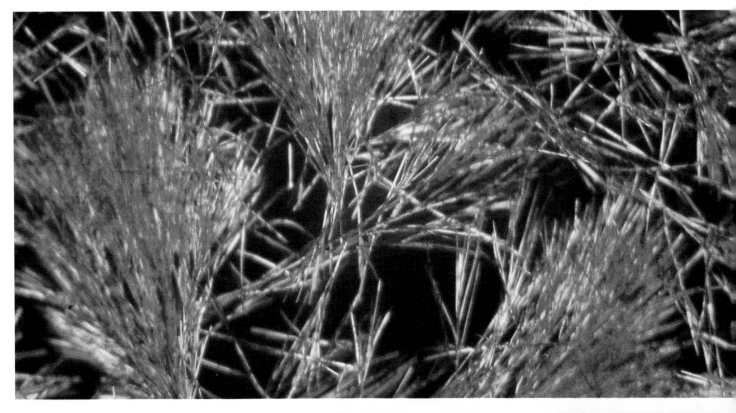

hormones. One of the most important of their actions is in prevention of blood clotting. Dr John Vane, a British pharmacologist, was awarded the 1982 Nobel Prize in medicine following his involvement in 1976 in the discovery of a prostaglandin released by arterial walls which prevented platelet clumping and thus clotting of blood. He described the substance, prostacyclin, as "one of the most potent (chemicals) known for preventing platelet aggregation."

Another common therapeutic use of prostaglandins is in helping women during childbirth. Here, the hormone is used as a drug to stimulate uterine contractions at full term when the birth of the baby is too slow. If given in midtrimester, the same action is used to stimulate abortion.

Although prostaglandins are generally "friendly," they do no favors to those suffering from arthritis and rheumatism. They have been found guilty of involvement in the inflammatory response associated with both of these conditions, and therefore can be treated with drugs such as aspirin

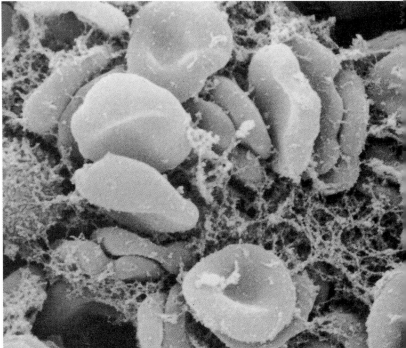

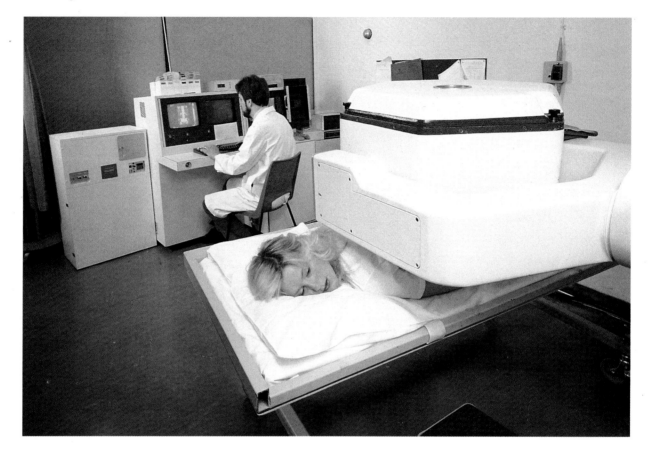

and indomethacin which inhibit the initial synthesis of prostaglandins.

Hormone Detection

The development of techniques to measure the concentrations of hormones has allowed scientists to increase their knowledge of the physiology of endocrine glands and endocrine disorders. Biological methods of measurement, known as bioassays, were the first to be used. These involve observing the effect of an unknown quantity of a hormone on a laboratory animal and comparing it with the effect of known concentrations of hormone. Such an assay is used to estimate concentrations of antidiuretic hormone (vasopressin), for example. An anesthetized rat which has drunk large amounts of water is given an injection of the test sample, for instance from a plasma sample. Other rats are given injections of known concentrations of vasopressin. The amount of excretion of urine

(diuresis) is measured thereafter in each case and the amount of vasopressin in the test sample can thus be determined.

The advantage of this type of assay is that it can be used to measure a hormone's concentration in terms of its biological activity. The technique is not, however, very accurate and the results are difficult to reproduce. There is also the cost and ethical problem of using laboratory animals and the time needed to complete such tests. For these reasons, scientists have in the past two or three decades developed more sophisticated analytical methods to estimate hormone concentrations.

Today the main method employed to measure hormone concentrations is radioimmunoassay, a technique devised first by Rosalyn Yalow in New York, working with Solomon Berson. Accurate to an amazing degree, the method was instrumental in the discovery of some of the hypothalamic hormones shortly afterward. It is used to investigate disorders that may be associated with endocrine dysfunction, thus helping physicians in their diagnosis and subsequent treatment. The test requires a "recognizer" substance or antibodies. To make antibodies, the particular hormone of interest is injected into an animal and can then act as an antigen to cause the manufacture of antibodies or proteins in the blood which combine with antigens to render them harmless. An antiserum, which contains "recognizers" or antibodies specifically against the hormone, can then be extracted from the animal and then used in a radioimmunoassay to determine the unknown hormone level.

The assay is carried out in a test tube in which a hormone sample of known concentration is labeled with a radioactive isotope and, along with the test sample, added to a known quantity of antibody obtained from the antiserum. The standard and test sample compete for binding sites on the antibody as if there were two keys and one keyhole. The free hormone and the hormone bound to the antibody can be separated using simple techniques. If the same amounts of labeled and unlabeled hormone are added to the antigen sample, then the same amount of labeled and unlabeled hormone should be bound. By carrying out the experiment with various known concentrations of labeled and unlabeled hormones, after the competition the free and bound portions of the sample can be counted for radiolabel and an analyst can compile a graph which can be used to estimate unknown concentrations. This technique does have limitations, however, such as the difficulty of preparing pure hormones for radiolabeling and obtaining very specific antibodies.

Hospital doctors may also need to know whether the rate of hormone production by an endocrine gland is sufficient, so that it is sending the right number of chemical messages to its target tissues. The production rate can be measured by labeling a hormone with a radioactive isotope, a known dose of which is given orally to a patient whose urine is then collected over a specified period of time. By separating out and measuring the amount of labeled and unlabeled hormone, a simple subtraction calculation of the difference determines the rate of that hormone's secretion by the endocrine gland in question.

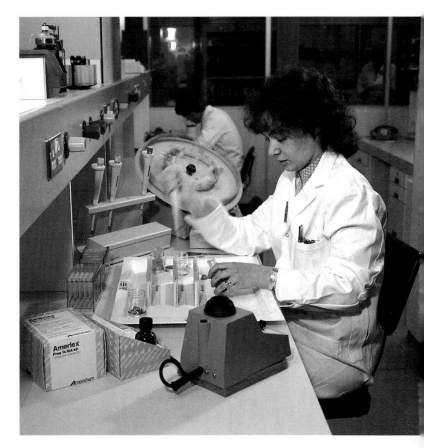

Testing blood samples for thyroid hormones is done by immunoassays, which involve labeling a hormone with isotopes, measuring further blood samples thereafter, calculating the difference between samples and so meanwhile measuring the gland's secretion of that hormone, thus determining its efficiency.

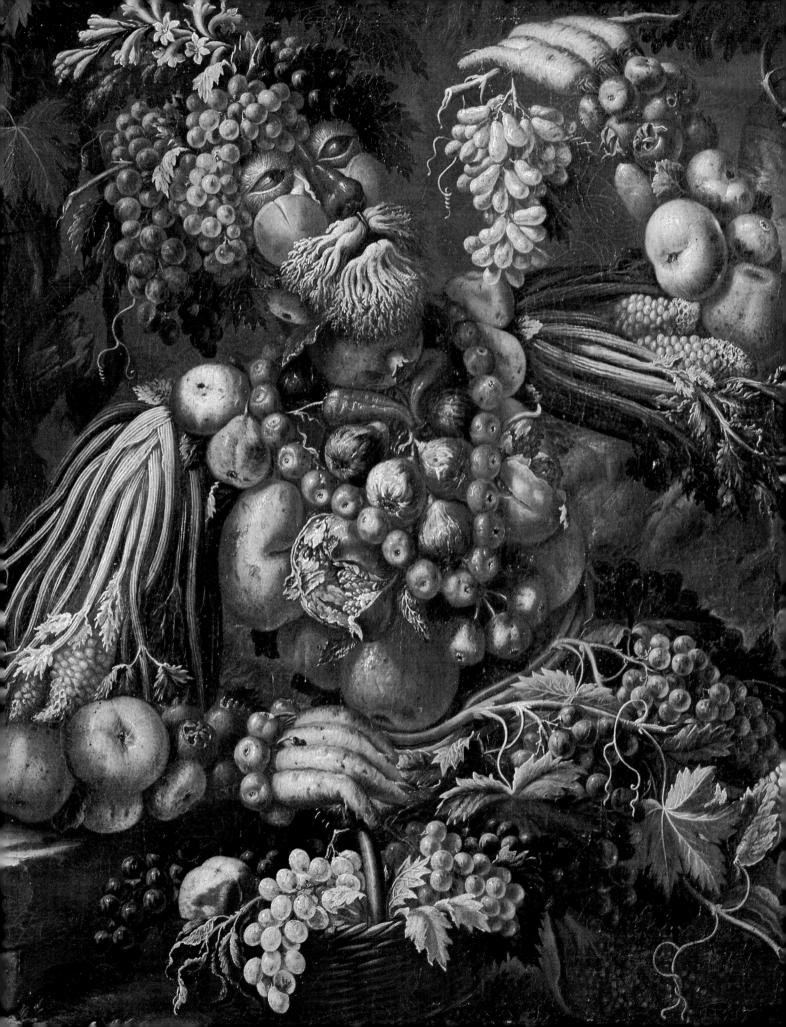

Chapter 5

Balancing the System

It is most unappealing, especially perhaps after a large meal, to reflect that we are all made of food — that people are what they eat. Yet, head to toe, every single cell in the human body is made up of nutrients derived from food. All human activity, from the purely unconscious processes of respiration and heartbeat, to composing a symphony or running a marathon, are fueled by food. From the moment of conception onward, the human organism needs food for growth and repair, and for energy to function at all levels.

The chemical conversion of food into building blocks or units of fuel, and the assembly of those building blocks into components of body tissue, is known as metabolism (from the Greek verb *metaballein*, meaning "to change"). There are two aspects to metabolism: catabolism, which is the breakdown of large molecules into smaller subunits (such as the degradation of complex carbohydrates into the simple sugar, glucose), and anabolism, which is the building up, the chemical synthesis, of new body tissue. In both its aspects metabolism is a never-ending process of change, mediated to a great extent by hormones circulating in the blood.

The first hint of the possible significance of hormones in metabolism came with the discovery that ushered in the science of endocrinology. Building on early work on digestion by pioneers such as the physiologist Claude Bernard, a Frenchman, and the legendary Russian Ivan Pavlov, two British physiologists, William Bayliss and Ernest Starling, came to recognize that there was something in the bloodstream governing the secretion of digestive juices. In fact the whole notion that chemical messengers influence events in parts of the body remote from their sites of origin can be said to date from the discovery by these two men in 1902 of a substance called secretin. Bayliss and Starling were able to show — correctly as it turned out — that secretin controls the production

The surreal composition by Giuseppe Arcimboldo, an Italian painter of the sixteenth century, aptly depicts the concept of people being what they eat. Food, broken down into its components, helps to form all the parts of our bodies and provides the energy for their efficient functioning, a process which is controlled to a certain extent by hormones.

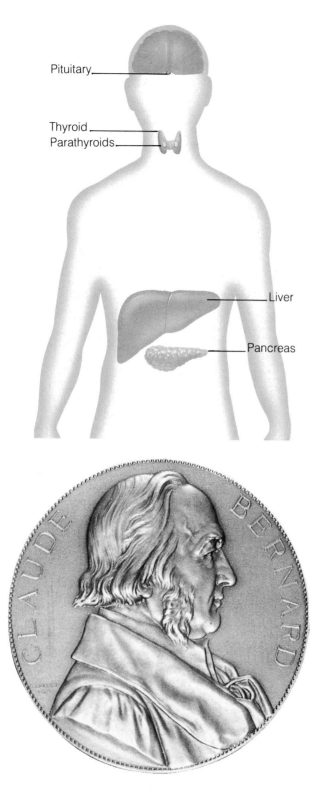

Pituitary

Thyroid
Parathyroids

Liver

Pancreas

Claude Bernard, a nineteenth-century French physiologist, first recognized the roles of the intestine and pancreas in digestion, although he did not know that hormones were involved.

The variety of food we eat (right) has only three main components — carbohydrates, fats and proteins — as well as vitamins and minerals. Their metabolism is controlled by the main endocrine glands (left).

of pancreatic juices. They called it a "hormone" and thus introduced the term into medical use.

In recent decades it has become apparent that hormones play a decisive role in maintaining the stable state known as homeostasis — the constancy of the body's internal environment despite external change. But the notion that good health depends on the preservation of some sort of internal balance is not a new one. The physicians of ancient Greece maintained that the human body was governed by its four "humors": blood, phlegm and black and yellow bile. Ill health, they believed, resulted from an excess of one of these humors.

More than two thousand years were to pass before the great investigator Claude Bernard combined the ancient concept of internal balance with a more up-to-date appreciation of physiological events. Bernard recognized that all vital functions are regulated through the interaction of tissues and are directed toward preserving the equilibrium of the internal environment, which he called the *milieu intérieur*. This key doctrine did not gain acceptance until it had been reiterated — and given the name homeostasis — by the Harvard physiologist W. B. Cannon, many years later.

So the purpose to which all metabolic change is directed is the preservation of homeostasis, the stable state. And it is as chemical taskmasters galvanizing the metabolic processes that hormones make their contribution to the cause.

The Process of Digestion

For an insight into the epic of metabolism, which continues to replenish tissues and fuel various body systems throughout our lives, it is pertinent to consider first the raw materials and the route they take from the dining table through the alimentary canal, through digestion with its assortment of acids and enzymes, to the ultimate sites of conversion either to a "building block" or to a source of energy within individual body cells.

There are three main organic components of food — carbohydrates, fats and proteins — each of which features rather differently in the body's overall energy scheme. Carbohydrates, for instance, which are found in all sugary and starchy foods, are a ready source of almost instant energy; they are the first substance to enter the bloodstream

96

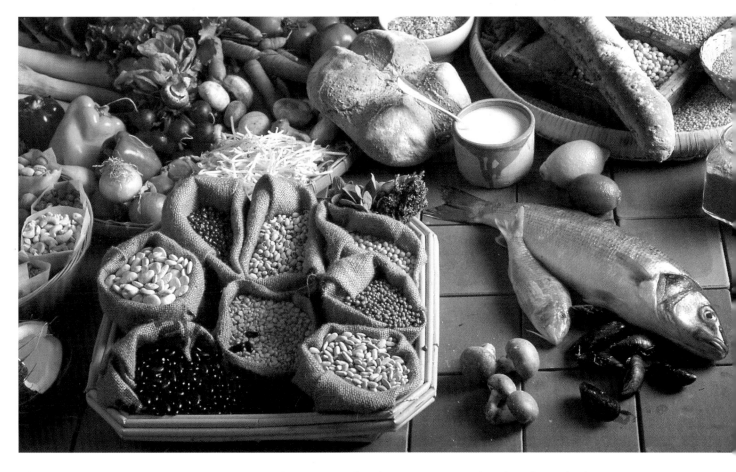

after a meal and are most readily converted into usable form — while fats and proteins are still being digested. Carbohydrate foods yield the simple sugar glucose, which is conveyed in the blood to every living cell. If not "burned" for immediate energy, glucose is stored in the liver and muscles as glycogen for short-term energy needs, and is converted into fatty tissues for intermediate and long-term energy needs. Carbohydrates make no contribution to body structure.

Fats in food are, on the other hand, slow to convert. Emulsified by bile salts, fats from all foods are broken down by enzymes into their component parts — fatty acids and glycerol — for uptake by the blood. Fats represent a more concentrated energy source than other foods, providing weight for weight more than twice the calorific value of proteins and carbohydrates. Excess fat is stored either in the liver or in fat cells which lie mostly under the skin. It is this insulating layer of fat which rounds out the body's contours and provides its prime energy bank, storing fuel for use in nutritionally lean times.

Protein, thirdly, is the basic material of living tissue, involved in every cell and every activity, from reproduction to defense. Proteins are large molecules — compounds of carbon, hydrogen, oxygen, nitrogen and, sometimes, sulfur — built up from chains of the 20 different subunits that are the amino acids. By continually re-ordering the amino acid sequences, the body can manufacture the many thousands of specific proteins needed for tissue formation, growth and repair. Because of its role in body building, protein — from foods such as meat, fish, cheese and eggs — is particularly important to a growing child, an expectant or nursing mother, and a manual laborer.

In addition to these organic components, a balanced diet must also provide small quantities of vitamins and minerals. The vitamins serve as hormonal substitutes that the body cannot manufacture, which act as vital reagents in a range of biochemical reactions. Minerals such as calcium, iron and phosphates are essential for the formation of bone, teeth and blood, for energy transfer, and for the functioning of enzyme systems; sodium and potassium feature throughout the cells and fluids. Finally, adequate fluid intake is important: the body carries out most of its functions in a fluid medium, and water, in one form or another, constitutes almost two-thirds of the body.

Before all these components of food can be

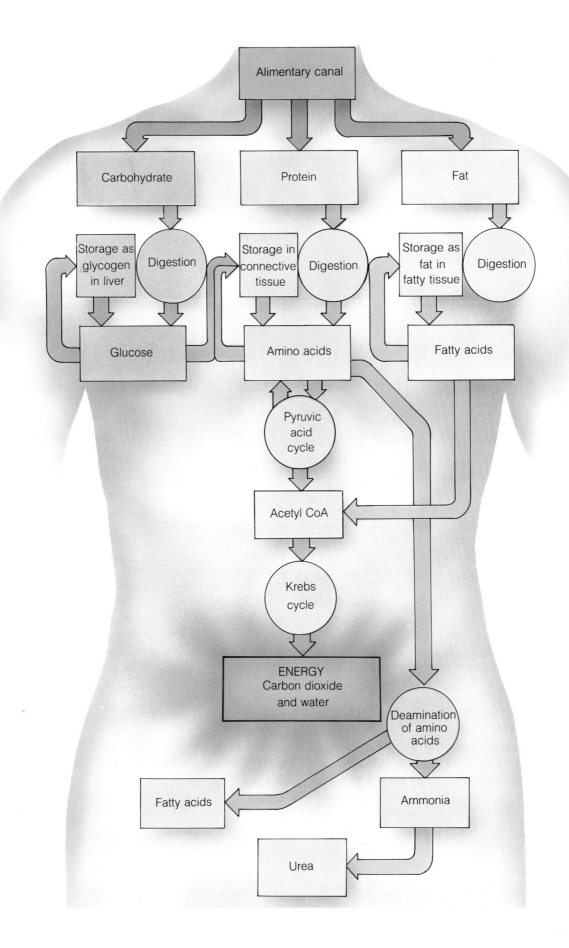

The digestion of food starts in the mouth. It is broken down all along the digestive tract and is stored in a variety of tissues, the waste being excreted. The metabolic processes involved provide fuel for energy.

The duodenum (below) secretes hormones which stimulate the pancreas and gall bladder to release enzymes and bile salts. These aid the absorption of food molecules by the villi of the intestine (bottom).

utilized by way of metabolic conversion, they must be digested and absorbed into the bloodstream. Digestion, which begins in the mouth through chewing together with the action of the salivary enzyme amylase, is really a process of fragmentation. It involves the use of physical forces (chewing) and chemical forces (enzymes and acids) to reduce food into soluble molecules small enough to be absorbed. The stomach secretes the foremost gastrointestinal hormone, gastrin, which triggers the release of digestive acid from the gastric glands. Blood flow to the stomach wall is also increased, enabling rapid absorption of a few substances, such as glucose, some salts and water, alcohol and certain drugs, which pass directly into the blood. But most of the stomach contents — by now reduced to a pulpy mass called chyme — are shunted into the intestines for further treatment.

The arrival of chyme in the first short loop of the intestine known as the duodenum signals the release of hormones which mobilize the pancreas to contribute its molecule-splitting enzymes and the gall bladder to release bile salts, which neutralize acids and assist in the emulsification of fats.

Through the wall of the intestine (studded with fingerlike villi which increase its absorptive surface) small molecules of food now pass into the bloodstream. Rendered into their constituent parts, carbohydrates are absorbed as simple sugars, fats as fatty acids and glycerol, and proteins as amino acids. These nutrients are carried from the intestine in the portal vein to the liver; fat molecules are also taken up by the milky-white lacteals in the intestine and make their way into the general circulation by way of lymphatic vessels; water and remaining salts are absorbed subsequently from food residues reaching the colon.

The liver has little to do with the digestion as such, beyond manufacturing and secreting bile (which is then passed to the gall bladder for storage). Even so, the largest and most industrious of the internal organs is central to the multitude of chemical processes which come under the general heading of metabolism. Receiving nutrients both from the portal vein (purveyor of the richest blood in the body) and the hepatic artery, the liver synthesizes glycogen, almost all the lipoproteins derived from fat, and many of the blood

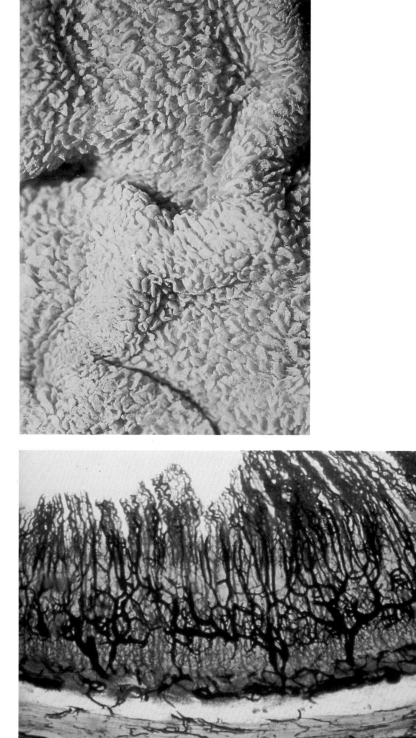

The stop-go system of traffic lights resembles the mechanisms of hormone release. A red light stops the traffic and a green light starts it just as a stimulus causes a hormone's secretion or inhibits it.

Fuel is energy which, in various forms, makes everything work. Burning coal provides the heat that fuels a steam engine and chemical reactions in the breakdown of glucose provide energy for the human body.

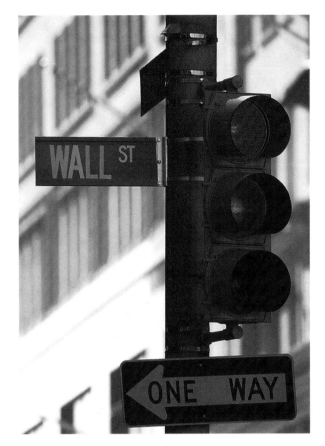

of delicate checks and balances on the energy resource as a whole.

Digestion at the Molecular Level

As in other life processes, the endocrine input in metabolism works on a stop-go basis: hormones are released into the bloodstream in response to one stimulus and inhibited in deference to another (the feedback mechanism). The primary function of the pancreatic hormone insulin, for instance, is the regulation of the universal body fuel, glucose, in the blood. A raised concentration of glucose in the blood, following a meal, triggers the release of insulin, prompting the uptake of glucose into the liver where it is converted to glycogen for storage.

When the glucose level in the blood returns to normal — within, say, one hour of the meal — the islets of Langerhans in the pancreas cease to secrete insulin. If this cut-off mechanism fails to operate, and insulin continues to flow into the circulation, the result is hypoglycemia, leading in the final extremes to collapse and coma. This is, in fact, the position of the severe diabetic who fails to preserve the critical balance between injected insulin and the intake of food. Conversely, diabetics can also suffer from too little insulin, which leads to a dramatic increase in the level of glucose and can culminate in diabetic coma.

The breakdown of nutrients has to do with changes at the molecular level and takes place in a watery environment, the so-called "internal sea" of interstitial fluid which bathes and supports both the cells and the fluid inside the cells.

Hormones involved in metabolism recognize their target tissues by means of hormone-specific receptors in the cell membrane. Once the connection has been made, the hormone and receptor may activate the appropriate metabolic reaction within the cell. Growth hormone, a product of the anterior pituitary gland, is an example of a hormone that works in this way. Alternatively, once the hormone cell wall receptor has been activated, a hormone may employ what is known as a "second messenger," cyclic AMP (cAMP). This substance initiates a reaction according to the instructions of the activated hormone, setting up a chain of events that ends with a specific chemical change.

As glucose is broken down in stages, energy is

proteins. It is also a storage depository for some nutrients, vitamins and minerals, and in particular for iron.

But principally the liver serves as a control gate in the energy cycle, filtering materials from the blood and storing them for release when the need arises. So, aside from its many other functions, the liver is the single most important organ in ensuring a constant supply of fuel for other tissues.

If all digested foods were allowed to circulate freely through the body, there would be a huge surplus to requirements. Instead, the absorbed components are utilized according to the needs of the moment, which may range from the simple requirements of the resting body — "idling" at what is known as the basal metabolic rate (BMR) — to the massive energy demands of strenuous exercise. It is in meeting these demands, and in controling metabolic output in general, that hormones exert their influence, operating a system

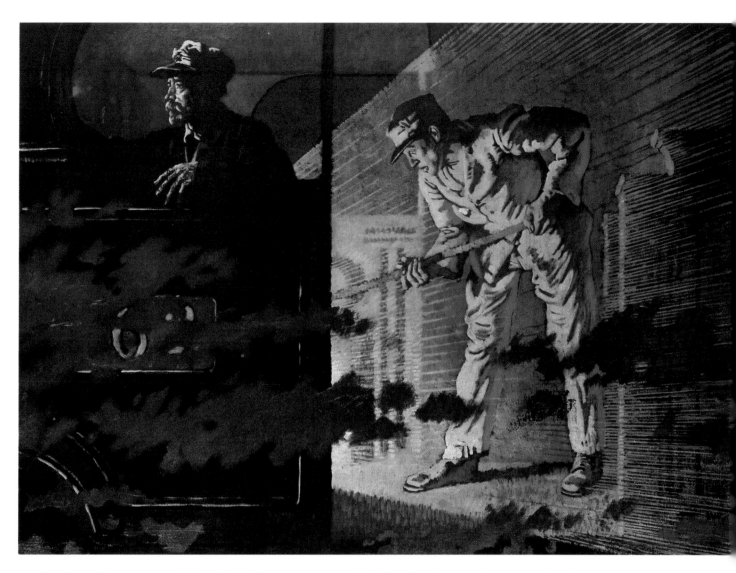

produced and is conserved in the high-energy compound adenosine triphosphate (ATP), the ubiquitous molecule which fuels many reactions throughout the body. Within the cell, ATP is metabolized with the help of the enzyme adenylate cyclase, which is generally found near the cell membrane. The hormone-receptor combination increases the activity of this enzyme, bringing about a rapid rise in cAMP which, in turn, activates a kinase enzyme. It is this little-understood but apparently multi-potent enzyme which acts as the starter for many different metabolic processes.

Carbohydrate Metabolism

The form of metabolism that deals with carbohydrates is of prime importance for restoring homeostasis after food is eaten. Carbohydrate metabolism mostly concerns glucose, the primary carbohydrate in the body. In the normal course of events, the body is usually subjected to mealtimes at which food is taken in, interspersed with periods of fasting. Yet despite this fluctuation, glucose levels in the blood are brought back to normal within an hour or so of eating and held in this steady state during the hours of fasting. This entire process is directed by the endocrine glands which compensate for change, secreting their hormones in response to the amount of glucose in the blood.

Carbohydrate metabolism ensures constant (and adequate) supplies of energy for all the vital body processes. While the liver cells immediately take up glucose absorbed from the intestines, some of this same fuel also makes its way into the general circulation. As soon as the increase in glucose is detected by the islets of Langerhans (in fact, while there is still food in the gut), these endocrine cells in the pancreas begin secreting insulin, the body's major sugar-lowering (hypoglycemic) hormone.

Known as the "hormone of plenty," insulin encourages the hoarding of glucose, stimulates its

Liver cells (below) synthesize glycogen from glucose and store it until energy is needed by the body's tissues. They also synthesize proteins and store nutrients such as iron and other minerals.

Cakes and cookies are a prime source of glucose, the most important carbohydrate. Its entry into the blood from the stomach induces the release of insulin, which speeds up its transportation to the liver.

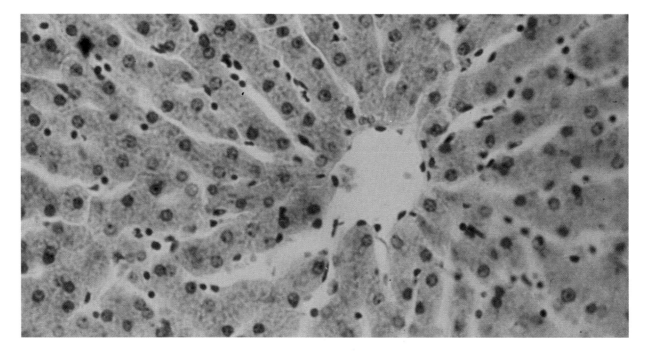

uptake by muscle cells and fat cells, and speeds up its rate of transport across the membranes of individual cells. Without the intervention of insulin, the concentration of glucose in the plasma would have to be ten to twenty times greater for it to be able to cross the cell membrane in sufficient quantity. In muscle, glucose not utilized immediately is converted to glycogen and stored for release in time of activity.

The hormone insulin is also active in the liver, where it encourages the synthesis of glycogen. In the form of glycogen, sugars can be stored and then converted back into glucose when the demand for energy increases. This is a biochemical equivalent of saving for a rainy day. In untreated diabetics, the capacity of the liver to make and store glycogen is impaired because of the reduction in or absence of naturally occurring insulin.

The islets of Langerhans in the pancreas also secrete a second hormone, glucagon, which counteracts many of the actions of insulin, operating on a negative feedback basis with its pancreatic colleague. Glucagon begins to take effect as the amount of glucose in the blood falls. In order to prevent hypoglycemia, the depletion of glucose in the blood, glucagon assists in providing readily available energy. Glucagon inhibits further conversion of glucose into glycogen and begins to mobilize the stores of glycogen in the liver so it can be converted back into glucose, for energy. In the liver cells, the enzyme adenylate cyclase is activated to begin the breakdown of glycogen and the formation of glucose from smaller molecules.

When blood glucose is low, most cells can depend on their stored supplies of glycogen for energy. A notable exception is the brain, in which the cells do not have adequate storage capacity. For this reason it is vitally important, in times of shortage, for glucose to be spared for the brain. The brain cells do not rely on insulin for the uptake of glucose, and can always obtain this fuel which is flowing freely in the circulation even when the concentration is too low for glucose to pass through cell membranes elsewhere in the body.

Unlike insulin, all the other hormones that influence carbohydrate metabolism are hyperglycemic — they increase the concentration of glucose in the blood. They come into play, for instance, following overnight fasting (when glycogen stores are much depleted) or during times of physiological stress — exercise, growth, illness — when the rate of fuel consumption goes up.

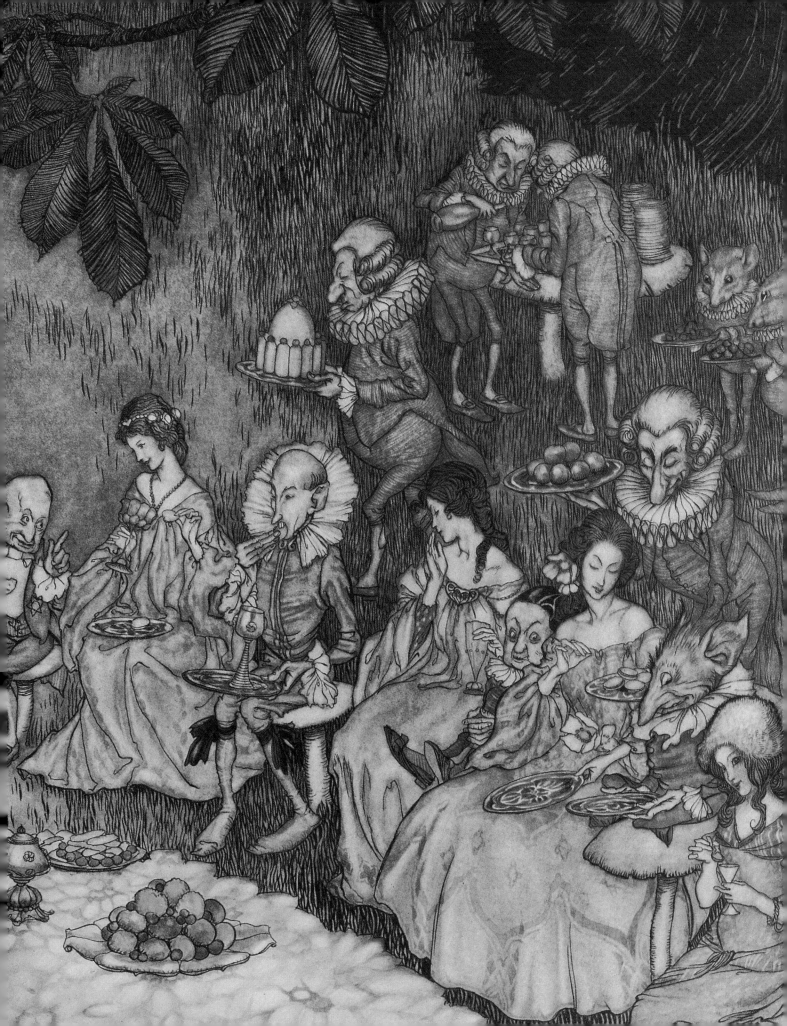

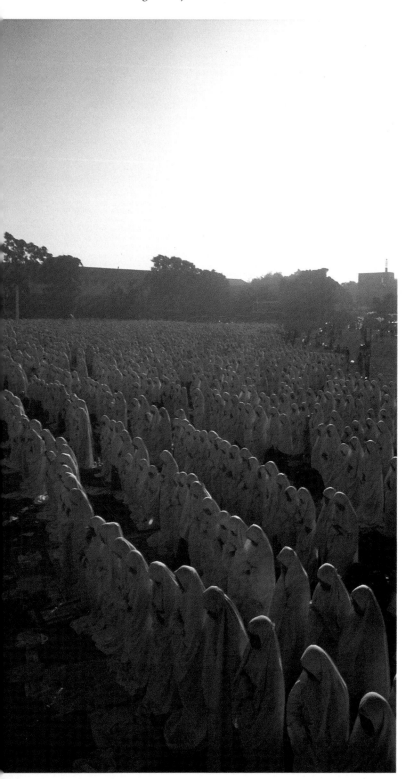

The Islamic celebration of Ramadan requires Muslims to fast in the daytime for a month. During a fast blood glucose level is low, so hormones are secreted which release glucose from its stores.

Growth hormone, secreted by the anterior pituitary and found in elevated concentrations in the blood during exercise or after a longer than usual overnight fast, has both glucose-increasing and glucose-saving functions. In its role as insulin antagonist, growth hormone decreases insulin's action on cell membranes, and thus helps reduce the capacity of these cells to absorb glucose. The blood glucose is augmented by the glucose output of the liver, further increasing the glucose concentration in the blood. Growth hormone also prompts glucose conservation in muscle and fatty tissues by making free fatty acids, another fuel, more readily available.

In the event of hypoglycemia induced by an excess of insulin, growth hormone is secreted to restore the balance by increasing the concentration of glucose. Secretion of the hormone is inhibited completely once there is excess glucose stored for consumption. This negative feedback mechanism is so dependable that it is used to test for acromegaly, the disorder which causes abnormal growth after maturity. Glucose is administered after a fast (when the glucose level is low and growth hormone is being secreted to restore the balance). If the addition of glucose fails to suppress growth hormone secretion within a short time, then a positive diagnosis of the disorder can be made.

Hormones secreted from the adrenal cortex which affect carbohydrate metabolism are the glucocorticoids, especially hydrocortisone (also known as cortisol). Hydrocortisone is also secreted in response to hypoglycemia, and helps maintain normal plasma glucose concentrations by encouraging the re-formation of glucose. It controls the conversion of glycogen, fatty acids and amino acids to glucose. During fasting, metabolic needs are met by the breaking down (catabolism) of protein in skeletal muscle and subsequent stripping of certain amino acids (deamination) in the liver where they are converted to glucose. The conversion and the formation of glucose are catalyzed by increased activity of several enzymes. The enzyme glucose-6-phosphatase in liver and kidney is necessary for glucose release into the bloodstream.

Epinephrine (also called adrenaline), the "fight or flight" hormone secreted by the adrenal medulla, is the body's first line of defense against

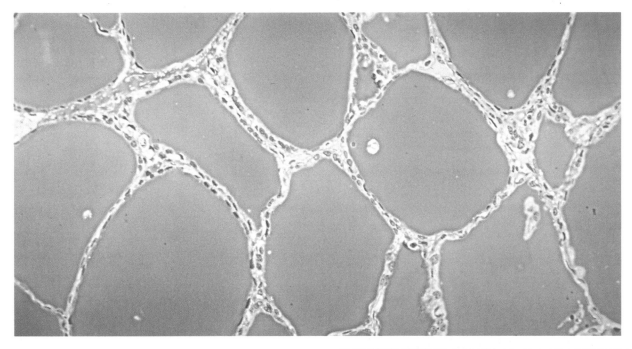

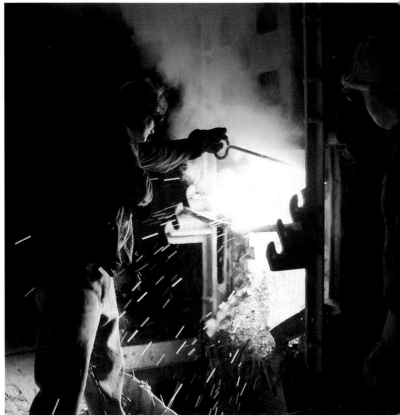

stress of all kinds. Among its effects is the mobilization of fuel reserves in all the body tissues in anticipation of rises in the metabolic rate. Epinephrine itself stimulates glucose transformation from glycogen in the liver and skeletal muscles by activating intracellular cAMP. The cAMP switches on the cascade of enzyme-catalyzed reactions which complete the conversion of glycogen to glucose.

Epinephrine also increases available glucose indirectly because it stimulates the release of adrenocorticotropic hormone (ACTH) by the anterior pituitary. This in turn, stimulates the release of hydrocortisone.

Although glycogen stores in skeletal muscle can be metabolized only on site, following release of epinephrine they can also be converted to the intermediary lactic acid and transported in this form to the liver for complete conversion to glucose. This mechanism also comes into play during vigorous exercise, and it is the gradual build-up of lactic acid in the muscles that determines how long a person can continue to exercise.

Whereas epinephrine is the hormone of crisis, provoking immediate response, the thyroid hormones act more slowly, and the metabolic changes

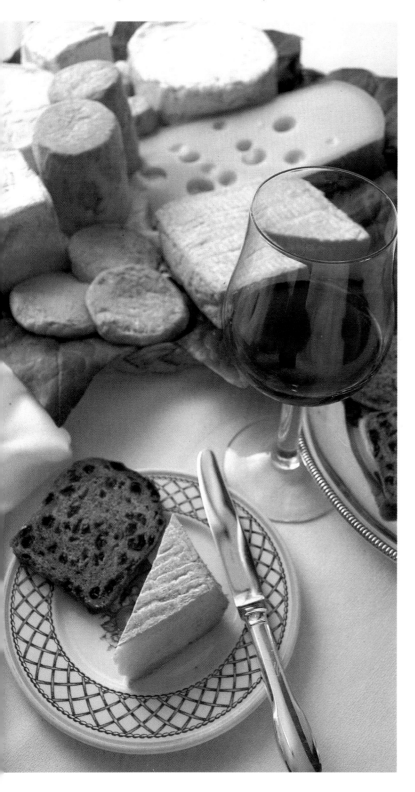

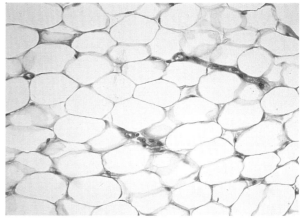

they induce may last for several days. Stressful conditions require the rate at which fuel is consumed — the basal metabolic rate (BMR) — to increase, the overall effect being that reserves of glycogen in the liver are quickly depleted. Thyroid hormones actually increase appetite and stimulate tissue-building activity while contributing to the breakdown of insulin, all of which lead to the availability of glucose in the body.

Fat Metabolism

Deposits of fat stored in adipose tissue are not simply a sign of good eating; they are life-sustaining, high-energy fuel supplies. Because only a limited amount of glycogen can be accommodated in the liver and skeletal muscles, one-third of any glucose passing through the liver is destined to be converted to fat and stored in this form. Insulin can stimulate the conversion of glucose to fatty acids in the liver, and can also promote the uptake of glucose by fatty tissue. Under the influence of insulin, the fatty acids are converted to storable fats in fat cells.

If fuel is needed, the first phase in the mobilization of stored fats is catalyzed by the enzyme hormone-sensitive lipase. The reaction produces glycerol and free fatty acids (FFAs), which enter the bloodstream and provide energy for cellular metabolism. Glucagon, growth hormone, glucocorticoids and epinephrine all stimulate the release of FFAs from fat cells.

Fatty acids provide a significant amount of energy for the muscles, and especially the heart.

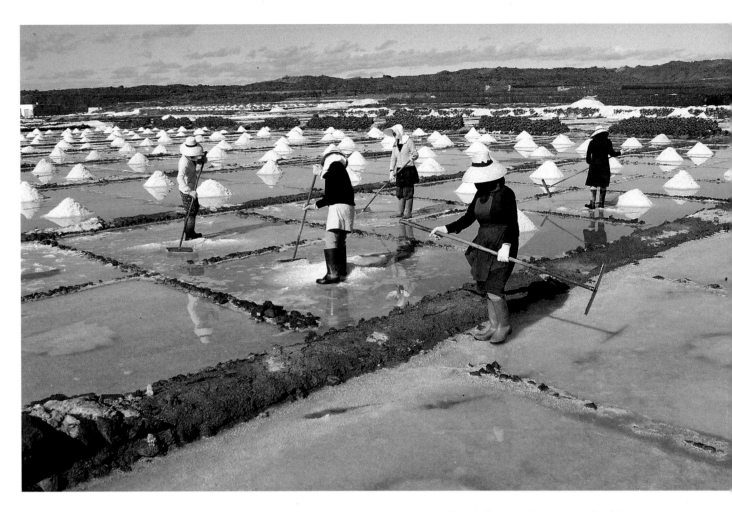

Their conversion to acetyl coenzyme A (acetyl CoA) and the subsequent metabolism of this substance yields more energy than does the metabolism of glucose. For this reason, fat is an even more highly concentrated form of stored fuel than glucose.

Protein Metabolism

The contribution of protein to the energy demands of metabolism is secondary to its role in tissue maintenance and renewal, where its metabolism is centered on the building up or stripping off of amino acids. Most amino acids can be converted into others by cellular enzymes. A few, known as essential amino acids, have to be derived from food because our bodies are unable to synthesize them. If needed, most amino acids can enter the metabolic cycle by being converted to glucose after initial breakdown (deamination) in the liver.

In the gastrointestinal tract, proteins are broken down into their constituent amino acids, which then enter the liver and join the circulating "amino acid pool." Appropriate amino acids are absorbed by cells as they are required for protein synthesis. The presence of insulin is critical for amino acid transport across the cell membrane, and this hormone stimulates protein synthesis.

Growth hormone is also significant for the absorption of amino acids in cells, by increasing the rate at which they are taken up. Thyroid hormone (T_4) is essential for protein synthesis, but normally occurs in only small quantities in the body. In higher concentrations, T_4 breaks down protein.

Salt and Water Metabolism

Endocrine secretions also play a critical role in the metabolism of inorganic compounds and in the most vital of homeostatic functions, the preservation of the body's water balance. Because most of the body consists of water — about ten gallons in a one hundred and fifty pound man — it is essential for this fluid volume to be maintained. Only about one per cent of water passes out of the body from the gut or by way of the kidneys; the remainder is reabsorbed. But on a hot day the body can sweat three gallons, and athletes exercising on a humid day can lose half a gallon an hour.

The key to the maintenance of fluid levels is the mineral sodium, gained mostly from common salt

Like other forms of metabolism, that of calcium is under hormonal control. When the blood calcium level is low, this state is communicated to the parathyroids via the hypothalamus and the pituitary. The parathyroids secrete parathormone, which induces the secretion of calcium from bone, and accelerates its absorption from the intestines and its secretion by the kidneys. When the blood calcium level exceeds the norm, the thyroid gland is stimulated to secrete calcitonin, which increases the rate of calcium deposition in bone, reduces its absorption from the intestine and increases excretion by the kidneys.

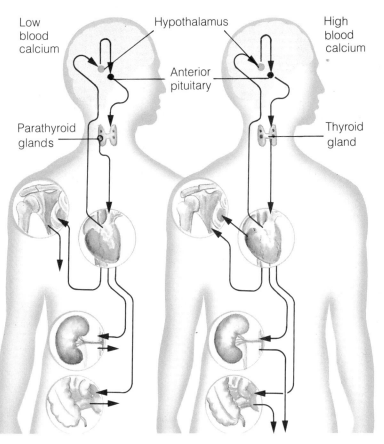

Low blood calcium

Hypothalamus

High blood calcium

Anterior pituitary

Parathyroid glands

Thyroid gland

kidneys. When sodium levels become depleted, water is lost and blood pressure falls. This potentially serious development is detected in the renal circulation, where the kidneys' response is to secrete the enzyme renin. This enzyme activates the hormone angiotensin which, in turn, stimulates the secretion of aldosterone. By reducing the permeability of the filter tubules in the kidney, aldosterone causes less water to be let out and at the same time alerts the hypothalamus to send out thirst messages. In this way, vasopressin, aldosterone and the hormone output of the kidneys work together to regulate the salt and water balance. If these controls were removed and the individual was unconscious, all fluid and salt would be lost from the body within a few hours.

Sodium also features in the constant exchange with potassium across cell membranes. The transaction is facilitated by means of the "sodium pump," a cellular device which expels sodium and assists the return of potassium into the cell. It is so important that it is one of the most energy-intensive activities in the body, accounting for a major part of the total fuel expenditure.

Calcium Metabolism

Calcium is a mineral mostly laid down in bone. The one per cent or so of free calcium in the body is essential for the normal functioning of the brain, nerves and muscles (including the cardiac muscle) and for blood clotting. It has also been suggested that calcium appears to act as a "third messenger" (after hormones and cAMP) in the chain-reaction of cellular metabolism.

Parathormone (PTH) from the parathyroid glands in the neck regulates the level of calcium in the blood very precisely, stimulating calcium release (along with phosphate) from bone as necessary. It also increases reabsorption of calcium and increases the rate of excretion of its mineral partner, phosphate, by the kidneys.

The key to adequate absorption of calcium in the gut is vitamin D, which is formed in the skin in the presence of sunlight. Vitamin D is then processed in two stages — first in the liver and then the kidneys — into the hormone known as 1,25-dihydroxycholecalciferol (or calcitriol). The synthesis of this hormone, which encourages the

in the diet. Since ancient times, salt has been recognized as essential to life but, even so, too much sodium in the interstitial fluid or blood vessels causes water to be leached out of the cells, resulting in cellular dehydration. The presence of too little sodium causes the cells to become waterlogged.

Thirst is not necessarily the result of dehydration, but may be caused by raised sodium levels in the body's extracellular fluids (including the blood). It is this fact that is communicated to the "thirst center" in the hypothalamus. We "feel thirsty" and increase our fluid intake — a very simple mechanism for restoring equilibrium. The hypothalamus also signals the posterior pituitary to release the antidiuretic hormone vasopressin, and this in turn acts to promote increased absorption of water by the kidneys, resulting in the production of a more concentrated urine.

Aldosterone, from the adrenal cortex, regulates the excretion of sodium and potassium from the

In times of dehydration (below) and starvation (right), hormones act to conserve the body's resources. The pituitary secretes water-retaining hormones and the body slows down to ration the remaining glucose.

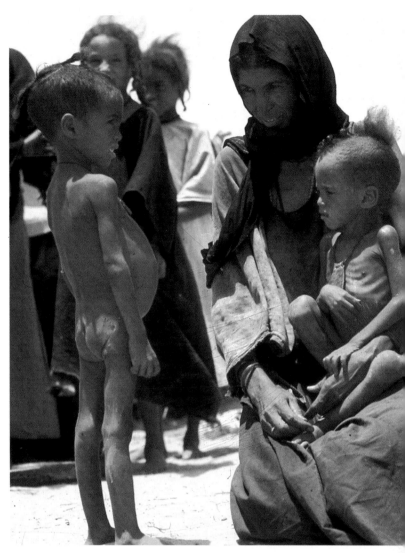

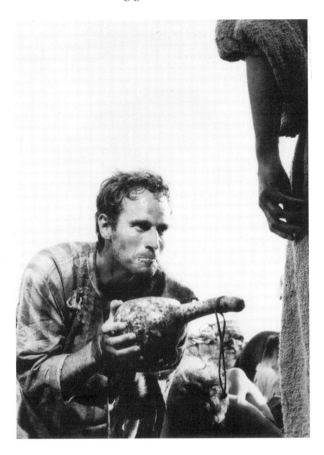

absorption of calcium from the gut, is stimulated by an increase in parathormone and a decrease in blood phosphate (a cry for calcium). Its synthesis is also stimulated by raised levels of estrogen, prolactin and growth hormone, ensuring increased uptake of calcium during the critical periods of pregnancy, lactation and growth.

Hormone Cooperation

It is when there is a threatened departure from homeostasis (due to factors arising from within the body or without) that the full range and elegance of hormone control of metabolism comes into play — the way in which different hormones work together to make good any destabilizing influence and ensure the best possible survival of the organism as a whole. A simple example is the smooth partnership of the adrenal medullary hormones, epinephrine and norepinephrine, in mustering the body's resources for emergencies.

But whereas the "fight or flight" response brings short-term changes, endocrine secretions are also involved in long-term adjustments geared to preserving homeostasis. Starvation, for instance, requires fundamental revisions in the fuel economy. Where there is prolonged deprivation of food, survival is guaranteed only by the hoarding of resources, and by mechanisms which eke out supplies of glucose and protein in particular. This is achieved by slowing down the body's systems. Growth hormone, for example, cuts glucose utilization to a minimum and mobilizes fat stores as a way of sparing the body from consuming its own protein structure. After the fat stores have been burnt off, the body "consumes" its muscles and the functioning of its systems, such as heart rate, slow down. The brain learns to adjust to low-grade fuel. In this way, so long as there is water available, it is possible for an average adult to survive for forty days or so without any solid food.

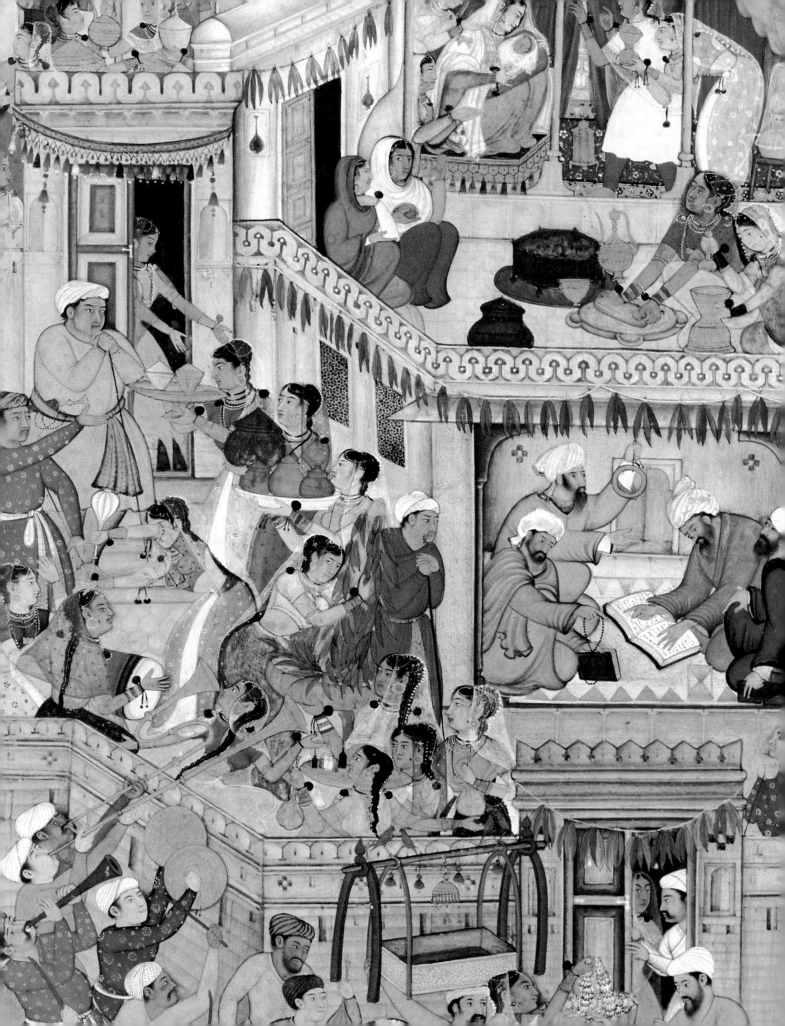

Chapter 6

Chemistry of Creation

The ancient Greeks believed that the sex of a child was determined by the strength of the "seed" from each parent. Father and mother both had within them male and female seeds, and the type of seed that prevailed determined the sex of the child.

That "girls will be girls" and "boys will be boys" is of course dictated by their genetic inheritance — the code held on one of the twenty-three pairs of chromosomes that are present in almost every nucleus of every cell of the body. When sperm and eggs are being formed, a special sort of cell division takes place so that they contain only one of each pair of chromosomes. When a sperm fertilizes an egg and both cells combine to form one cell the correct number of chromosomes is reinstated.

The arrangement of the sex chromosomes is such that all the eggs a woman produces have an X chromosome, whereas a sperm has either an X or a Y chromosome. When a sperm with a Y chromosome pushes its way into the egg and tips out its twenty three chromosomes, each combines with a partner from the twenty-three chromosomes in the nucleus of the egg; twenty three pairs are thus formed, one of which will be an XY pair. The fertilized egg is destined to become a boy. On the other hand, if it is an X-containing sperm the sex chromosome pair will be XX, and a girl develops.

Although the eventual sex of a child is therefore predetermined at conception, it is really the hormones that direct the development of the sexual features. In fact, to be more precise, it is the male sex hormone that nudges a forty-day-old XY fetus into developing the characteristics of a male. Until this stage in fetal development the small clusters of cells destined to form the reproductive system are identical in both male and female fetuses. Internally they are the same: there are two undifferentiated gonads and two sets of ducts. The external genitalia also look the same: a bud protruding from a slit with a swelling on either side.

High-spirited revelers in northern India rejoice with music and dancing at the birth of Mogul Emperor Akbar's second son Murad, in 1570. After nine months of finely controlled nurturing in the mother's womb, the traumatic experience of delivery is the final stage in the wondrous creation of a new life.

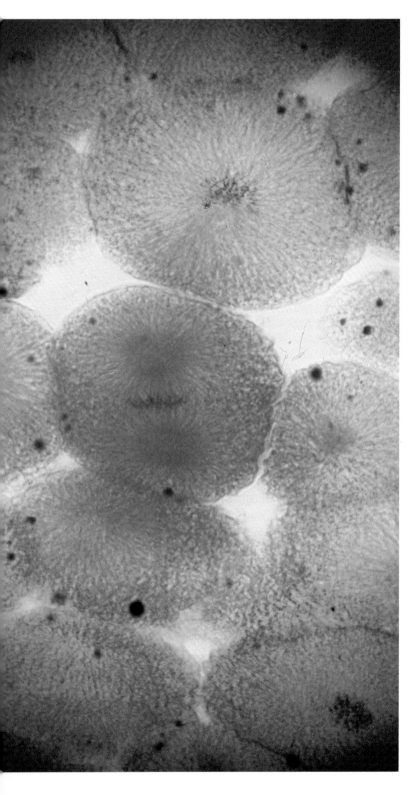

Essential to life, meiosis is the process by which egg and sperm cells are formed. A cell divides to produce two new cells (either eggs or sperm), each with one-half of the "parent" cell's chromosomes.

It is at this point that the genetic inheritance has an effect, for it is the presence of a Y chromosome that in some way switches on the development of the testes from the primordial cells of the undetermined gonad. The turning-point has been reached, and the growing testes begin to release the hormone testosterone, which causes the system to form male sex organs. One set of ducts regresses; the surviving pair grow to become the vas deferens and seminal vesicles. Externally, the "bud" becomes the penis, and the two swellings fuse and form the scrotum into which the testes later descend. Without testosterone the male ducts and external genitalia just do not develop. Instead, the other set of ducts form the Fallopian tubes, the uterus, cervix and vagina. And externally the small bud stays as the clitoris and the two swellings become the labia. The slit between them does not close, and both the uretha and vagina open into it.

There is an interesting, although very rare syndrome, which shows just how important testosterone is in establishing male development. This is the testicular feminization syndrome which arises when a genetically male fetus (XY) is unable to respond to the testosterone released by the growing testes. Consequently, the male external genitalia do not develop, and a baby with the appearance of a girl (but genetically male) is produced. This syndrome can remain completely undetected until adolescence, when the absence of menstruation may be questioned. Then it is discovered that "she" is genetically male, but has external female genitalia, with a vagina which ends blindly. There are small, underdeveloped testes and, of course, no ovaries.

The Events of Puberty

When babies are born, their ovaries or testes are not really working. They do not produce gametes (sperm or ova), but do release very small amounts of steroid hormones — mainly testosterone in boys and estrogens in girls. The pituitary gonadotropins, luteinizing hormone (LH) and follicle-stimulating hormone (FSH), are also released under the influence of the hypothalamic releasing hormone, but again at very low levels. The whole system is latent, just quietly running in neutral as though waiting for the green light signal to go.

The signal comes when the body is mature enough for reproduction — it is the time of puberty when reproductive capability is achieved. Just what stimulates the gonads into activity is not really known.

One hypothesis to explain the onset of puberty is that the negative feedback effects of puberty and testosterone on the release of luteinizing hormone and follicle-stimulating hormone become less effective — more gonadotropins are produced, and the gonads are stimulated. But whatever the exact mechanism, it seems that the ultimate outcome is an increase in the frequency of the hormone signal from the hypothalamus that reaches the pituitary gland.

The onset of puberty is obvious. Pubic hair begins to grow; girls start to develop breasts and their hips widen; and boys grow stubble on their chin and their voice deepens. It is also a time when there is a sudden growth spurt, and a change in the composition of the body. Girls lay down more fat than boys, so when adulthood is reached, women generally have proportionally more body fat than men, whereas men have about one and a half times the lean body mass of women. Men also have many more muscle cells, which accounts for the greater physical strength of males.

All these physical changes are caused by the surge of sex hormones — estrogen and testosterone — which stimulate the development of what are termed secondary sex characteristics. It commonly happens earlier in girls and the first menstruation (or menarche) usually occurs between ten and sixteen years of age. Boys tend to reach puberty between fourteen and eighteen, although there is no single obvious external sign when this happens.

Living standards, and hence nutrition, seem to be important in the attainment of puberty. As nutritional standards have improved during this century, the average age for puberty has decreased. In the United States the mean age for menarche in 1900 was fourteen years, but by 1960 this figure had dropped to below thirteen years.

The ancient Chinese took a great interest in the philosophy of numbers which influenced their ideas about medicine, and within that field about the differences in male and female development.

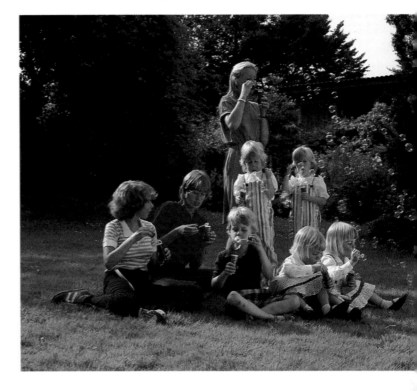

Female life, they thought, was dominated by the number seven. Teeth grow at seven months and seven years, puberty and the menarche begin at fourteen and the menopause at forty-nine. For men the dominant figure was eight, so teeth appeared at eight months and eight years; puberty occurred at sixteen and the male decline at sixty-four. Later in history (A.D. 1593), Ch'eng Ta-Wei even postulated a mathematical formula for establishing the sex of a child during intrauterine life!

Sometimes puberty occurs abnormally early, and children below the age of nine or ten years of age can reach full sexual maturity. This generally happens because the hypothalamus starts secreting the gonadotropin-releasing hormone inappropriately early, and the gonads are induced into an early maturation. This causes true precocious puberty, whereas another type of hormone abnormality stimulates early development of the secondary sex characteristics but the gonads do not mature and individuals so affected remain infertile. Such development may occur either as a result of a tumor or when high levels of steroid hormones are secreted from the gonads themselves or from the

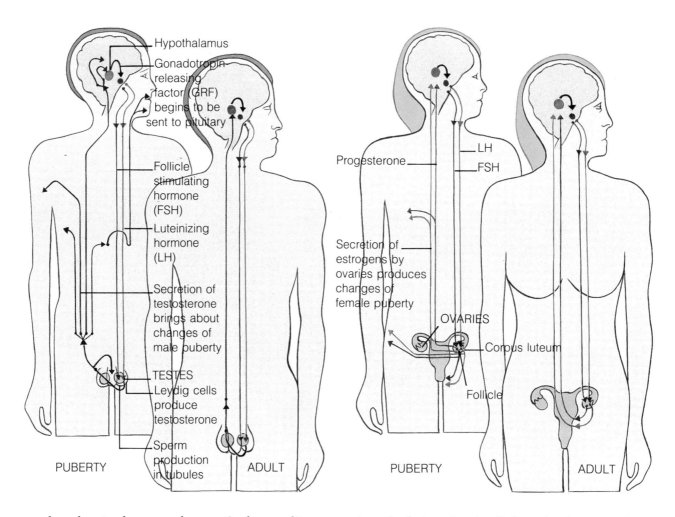

Hypothalamus

Gonadotropin releasing factor (GRF) begins to be sent to pituitary

Follicle stimulating hormone (FSH)

Luteinizing hormone (LH)

Secretion of testosterone brings about changes of male puberty

TESTES

Leydig cells produce testosterone

Sperm production in tubules

PUBERTY

ADULT

Progesterone

LH

FSH

Secretion of estrogens by ovaries produces changes of female puberty

OVARIES

Corpus luteum

Follicle

PUBERTY

ADULT

adrenal cortex because of a genetic abnormality.

One of the great systematic physiologists of the eighteenth century, the Swiss Albrecht von Haller (1708–1777), documented a series of cases of precocious puberty and tried to dispel the idea that these poor children were merely freaks created by supernatural influence. One particularly sad, and extreme, case history of his was of a Swiss girl who started menstruating at the age of two. At eight she became pregnant by her uncle, and nine months later she delivered a stillborn child.

Male and Female Hormones

Although testosterone is generally thought of as the male hormone, it in fact represents just one of a number of hormones generally called androgens, all of which contain nineteen carbon atoms in their molecular structure. However, testosterone is the most potent of the androgens, and is the one secreted in the highest concentration from the testes. Estrogens such as estradiol, estrone and estriol are made from testosterone and other androgens, but these female steroids differ from the male hormones in that they have eighteen carbon

atoms in their molecules. So by a simple conversion of testosterone to estrogen, all the masculinizing effects of testosterone can be neutralized, and the development of male characteristics suppressed. Even in adulthood these steroids can have powerful actions on sexual appearance. High concentrations of androgens tend to masculinize women, whereas estrogens have feminizing effects on men. For obvious reasons such effects are normally undesirable, although this form of treatment is used in conjunction with sex-reversal operations and the treatment of some tumors.

After puberty the reproductive years begin, and the steroids manufactured in the testes or ovaries help to maintain the output of sperm or ova and to regulate the pituitary output of gonadotropic hormones. The hormonal control of fertility therefore involves the brain through the hypothalamus which releases gonadotropin-releasing hormone, the pituitary gland which releases LH and FSH, and the gonads.

Many features of this control system are similar in men and women but women show cyclical changes in their fertility, whereas men have no

114

At puberty, there is an increase in gonadotropic secretions from the pituitary, and a rise in estrogen or testosterone levels. The gonadotropic signal is eventually powerful enough to start production of eggs or sperm.

Cold climates affect the average age at which girls begin to menstruate. Lapp girls start menstruating notably later than girls living in temperate climates, where the average age of onset is 13 years.

cyclical pattern. The ovaries normally produce between them just one ripe egg a month. In the testes about 200 billion sperm are produced every day. Not all survive — but even so, such significant production would have been a cause for amazement to the ancient Greek philospher Aristotle (384–322 B.C.), who believed that the testes were merely weights holding down the spermatic cords!

Sperm are produced in the seminiferous tubules of each testis, under the influence of FSH and testosterone. In between these tightly packed tubules are small cells, called Leydig or interstitial cells; it is these cells which produce the testosterone in response to the other gonadotropin, LH. Testosterone not only maintains the constant production of the sperm, but it also has important feedback effects on the brain. This feedback loop helps to stabilize the system so that the hormones involved in controlling the testes are kept at a correct and steady level.

Exactly what the influence of testosterone is on sexual behavior, libido and male aggressiveness, has long been questioned. Looking at the mammalian evolutionary tree it is possible to see that many lower mammals are totally dependent on testosterone for sexual activity. Removal of the testes of, say, a mouse or a ram results in the male animal being totally disinterested in females. It is not true of humans; a glimpse back in time shows that castrated men — eunuchs — were perfectly capable of sexual attraction and intercourse but only if they were castrated after puberty. In fact, in the society of imperial Rome, eunuchs were actively sought out by women because there was no fear of pregnancy. But it is true to say that castration does dull libido or sexual desires, even if it does not extinguish the flame completely — which is, of course, why castration was practiced on such a large scale, particularly on slaves, in the priesthood of various cults and on male attendants of a harem.

The Menstrual Cycle

Nearly two thousand years ago, Hippocratic writers documented that certain times of the menstrual cycle were "propitious for conception," and conversely the rhythm method was one of the techniques advocated for controlling fertility. If

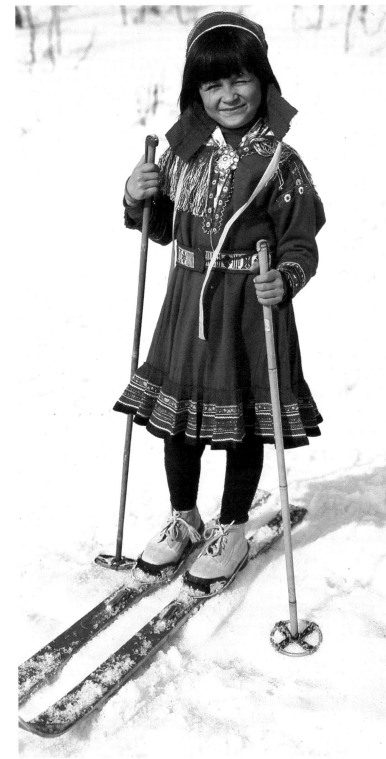

115

Male fallow deer show aggression in a horn-locked combat. Increased testosterone secretion during the mating season drives the males to compete for females, which ensures that only the strongest procreate.

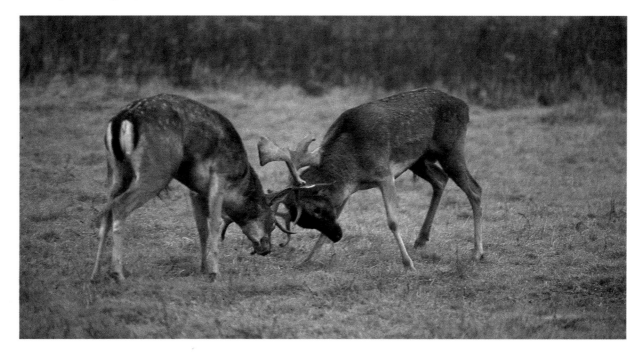

conception was required, intercourse was set for the tenth day after the beginning of menstruation. This certainly sounds like a very modern arrangement, and the Greeks were just about right, of course, but they had no idea why or how these menstrual cycles occurred. Today we know that it is due to hormonal interplay between gonadotropin secretion and the feedback effects of ovarian steroids on the hypothalamus and pituitary.

Starting at the beginning of the cycle—which is generally taken to be the first day of menstrual bleeding—the circulating levels of estrogen, and of the other major ovarian hormone, progesterone, are very low. The negative feedback effects of these hormones is minimal, which allows the release of the hypothalamic releasing hormone and the LH and FSH to increase. They then stimulate the growth of a few eggs otherwise dormant in the ovary.

The eggs are surrounded by a sac of cells, and some of these minute packages begin to grow when they receive the gonadotropin signal. The egg enlarges, the follicular cells around it divide and form a complex capsule, and eventually the mature egg is suspended from the inner layer of follicular cells in a fluid-filled cavity (the antrum).

While the follicles are developing they release increasing amounts of estrogen, which has a negative feedback effect on the release of gonadotropin. Toward mid-cycle, however, several things happen. Most of the ripening follicles begin to regress, and are absorbed and forgotten forever. Usually only one (but occasionally more) reaches the right stage of maturity at the right moment to respond to the gonadotropin signals; this favored follicle enters into the final stage of development, and prepares itself for ovum release. At about the same time, the estrogen levels in the blood rise to a critical point. Suddenly the estrogen no longer tends to suppress gonadotropin release — quite the opposite. In some unknown way the negative feedback effects on the hypothalamic-pituitary axis become positive, and there is an explosive surge of luteinizing hormone secretion which causes the ripe follicle, bulging from the surface of the ovary, to burst open. The egg, surrounded by a protective layer of follicular cells, is released and wafted into a Fallopian tube. Ovulation has occurred, and conception can take place.

Ovulation, which normally occurs around the fourteenth day of the menstrual cycle, marks the end of the follicular phase, and as the empty follicle

A female bodybuilder (below) cannot enlarge her muscles as a man can because women's bodies lack testosterone — production of which, in women, can cause abnormal growth of facial hair (right).

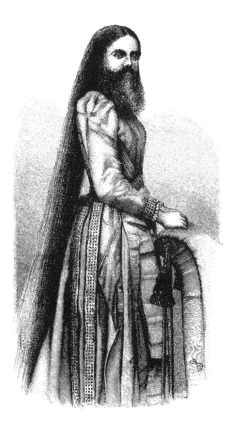

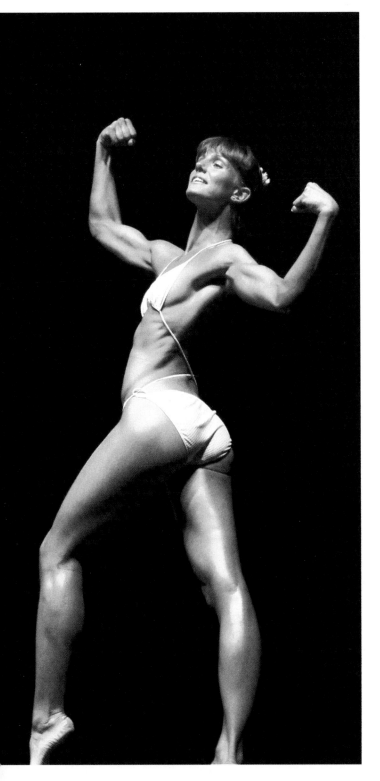

collapses in on itself, the luteal phase of the cycle begins. It is called the luteal phase because the collapsed follicle forms a "corpus luteum" — a solid mass of cells synthesizing estrogens and relatively high concentrations of progesterone. The luteal phase is thus dominated by progesterone, which inhibits gonadotropin secretion and helps build up the lining of the womb, preparing it for implantation of the conceptus if fertilization should take place. One clinical marker for ovulation is to measure the progesterone concentrations in the blood during the second phase of the cycle. If ovulation has not occurred, there is no luteal formation and the progesterone levels remain low. Another marker of ovulation is a slight rise in basal body temperature.

The cycle ends with luteolysis. This occurs when the corpus luteum breaks down and stops manufacturing estrogen and progesterone. The cycle is over, and the withdrawal of steroids allows the gonadotropins to rise and start off the maturation of another set of follicles. A new cycle begins. At the same time the lining of the womb (the endometrium) is no longer supported by the steroid hormones and it begins to fall away. The tiny spiral arteries which have grown up into the

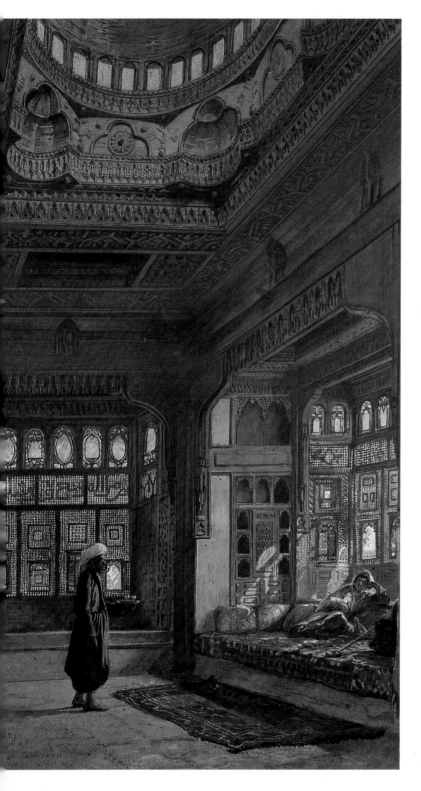

Attended by a eunuch, a member of a harem relaxes in an Egyptian palace. Throughout history, eunuchs — men who have had their testicles removed — were employed as prized guardians of a ruler's many wives.

lining are broken — and thus the bleeding of menstruation. It happens only in female humans, apes and Old World monkeys; in other mammals the lining of the womb is not shed but instead is resorbed and replaced by a new lining. There is therefore no bleeding and shedding of the endometrium.

Menstruation and Science

The process of menstruation has aroused the interest of physicians and biologists since antiquity. Its connection with the length of the lunar cycle (hence the term *menses*) was always obvious, but its connection with the ovaries and ovulation was not really made until the end of the nineteenth century.

From the time of Hippocrates, menstruation was thought to be a sort of detoxification process of a form of blood-poisoning that women suffered. Women were therefore unclean during this period, and ancient priestesses were banned from carrying out their religious duties during menstruation. In the Old Testament, a menstruating woman was regarded as "unclean." Among some cultures and religious sects this view has persisted right up to the present day.

The first scientific account about the effects on menstruation of removing the ovaries was reported by the English surgeon Percivall Pott in 1775. He performed the operation on a young woman to cure an "ovarian hernia" and noted that it was followed by shrinkage of the breasts and cessation of her menses. This was an important observation, but it seems to have been totally ignored until a student working in Edinburgh noticed Pott's report and commented on it in his doctoral thesis (1794). He suggested that menstruation was caused by a peculiar condition of the ovaries which served as a source of excitement of the blood vessels of the womb. Toward the end of the nineteenth century ovulation was connected with menstruation, but still the causes remained elusive. Only at the beginning of this century did scientists really begin to understand that the ovaries were necessary for ovulation, and in the United States in 1923 and 1924 Edgar Allen and Edward Doisy published two papers about an ovarian hormone. They had isolated "oestrin" from the ripening follicles, and their experiments marked the beginnings of a

The ovulatory cycle starts with about five days of menstruation, during which the endometrium is shed. The endometrium is repaired under the stimulus of estrogen secreted by ovarian follicles in response to follicle-stimulating hormone. By day twelve, one follicle begins to mature. The release of luteinizing hormone at mid-cycle, on about day fourteen, discharges the ovum into a Fallopian tube and initiates the production of progesterone from the collapsed follicle (corpus luteum). If by day twenty-six fertilization has not occurred, the ovum dies, the corpus luteum ceases hormone production and the cycle restarts.

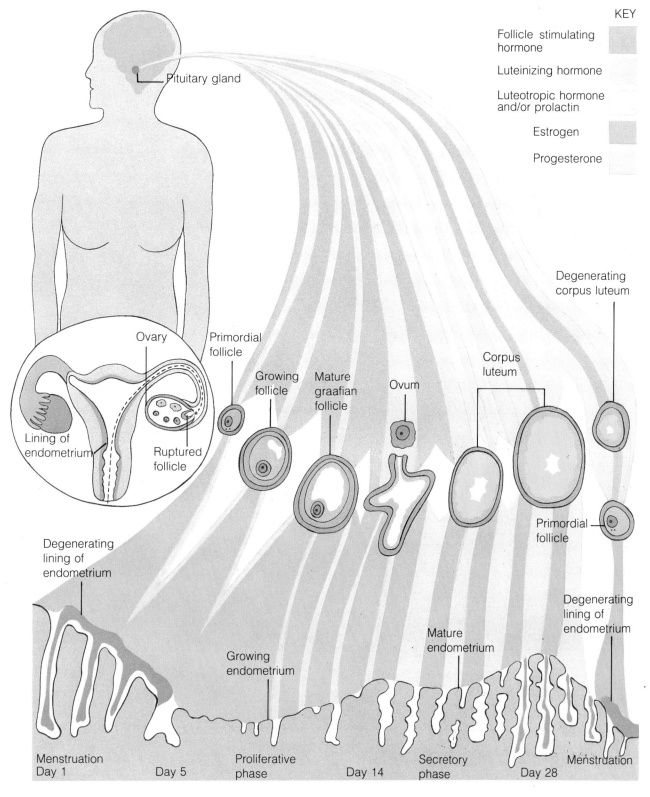

KEY

Follicle stimulating hormone

Luteinizing hormone

Luteotropic hormone and/or prolactin

Estrogen

Progesterone

Pituitary gland

Degenerating corpus luteum

Ovary

Primordial follicle

Corpus luteum

Growing follicle

Mature graafian follicle

Ovum

Lining of endometrium

Ruptured follicle

Primordial follicle

Degenerating lining of endometrium

Degenerating lining of endometrium

Mature endometrium

Growing endometrium

Menstruation Day 1

Day 5

Proliferative phase

Day 14

Secretory phase

Day 28

Menstruation

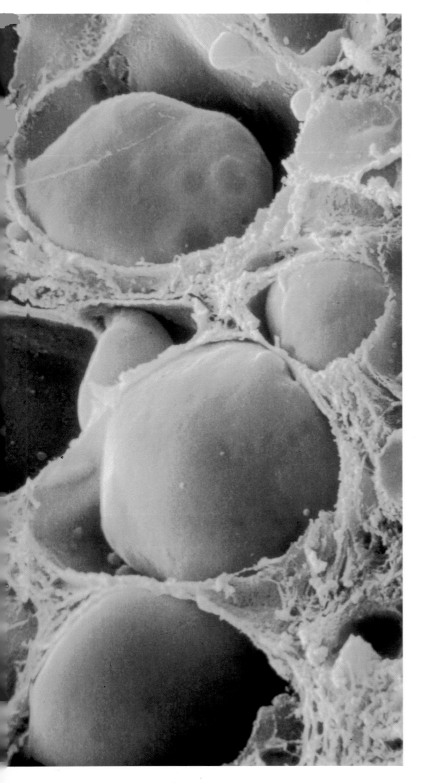

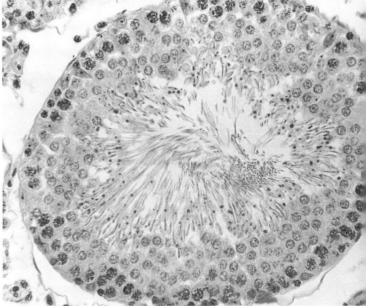

new era in reproductive endocrinology, and the discovery of the role of hormones in controlling the cycle of fertility.

Contraception

Methods of preventing conception have been practiced since prehistoric times, although in many early cultures it is unlikely that contraceptive methods were widely used; fertility was important, and barren women were a source of worry and shame. But when social ethics and the laws of a culture did not demand high fertility rates, contraception was practiced. Methods recorded throughout history for preventing pregnancy could fill several volumes. They range from barrier methods through oral potions, to substances and lotions placed in the female vagina or on the male organs. Ground cabbage blossoms, ivy leaves spread with honey, or the bark of a white poplar tree mixed with a kidney of a mule, are just three weird and wonderful examples of literally thousands of contraceptive concoctions that have been prescribed through the ages.

When Margaret Sanger and Marie Stopes opened the first birth-control clinics in the United States and in England during the first part of this century, they had only the barrier methods of contraception

There is a long-held belief that the menstrual cycle is in some way regulated by the moon, whose pervading influence is depicted in this Japanese painting. The length of the cycle is close to 29.5 days, a synodic month. Further evidence to suggest that the synodic month is biologically significant comes from the fact that the average duration of pregnancy is, in humans, nine 29.5-day synodic months (266 days).

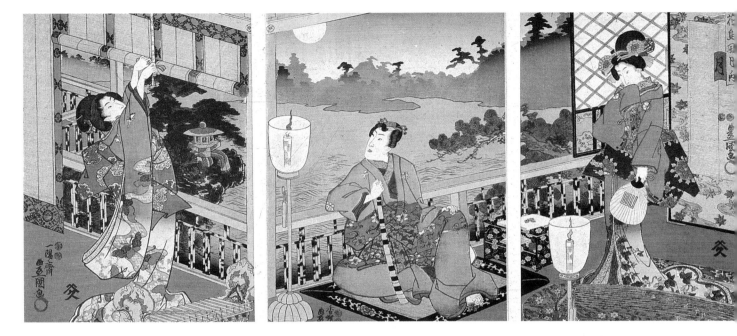

— the condom and the Dutch cap — which they could promote for safe contraception. The Pill was to come later, after the first large-scale clinical trials were carried out in South America in 1956.

Dr Gregory Pincus has been called the "Father of the Pill" because of his work which led to the development of the oral steroid contraceptives. He knew that progesterone output was increased at the time a fertilized egg implants itself into the lining of the uterus, and that this prevented the release of more ripe eggs. So he fed rabbits progesterone and found that it stopped them from getting pregnant. An experiment was made on women in 1952, and four years later a synthetic substance, norethynodrel, was eventually manufactured. Clinical trials were soon underway.

Over the years, new types of synthetic steroids have been developed. There are continued efforts to find ways to reduce the actual dosage of the hormones because in the long term they may have detrimental effects, particularly regarding tumor growth and on the circulatory system and heart. Nevertheless, their high efficacy as a means of contraception, and their obvious advantages over barrier methods, have maintained their popularity, especially with younger women. For women approaching their forties, however, and particular-ly those who are smokers, it is strongly recommended that they discontinue using oral contraceptives containing estrogen, because of the increasing risks of cardiovascular disease.

In essence, oral contraceptives work to maintain relatively high levels of circulating steroid hormones, causing negative feedback effects on the hypothalamus and pituitary, which then decrease secretion of LH and FSH. Ovulation and implantation are thus inhibited. There are two main types of oral contraceptives: the combined pill, which contains both estrogen and progesterone, and the progesterone-only pill. The combined pill is taken for 21 days, followed by a placebo or a pill-free week during which time menstrual bleeding occurs as a result of the withdrawal of the steroids. The progesterone-only pills are not taken cyclically but continually and, although they do inhibit ovulation, they are less reliable in this respect than the combined estrogen-progesterone pill. Instead, they rely mainly on their effects on the endometrium of the womb which tend to inhibit implantation of the conceptus. Menstrual bleeding does occur with the progesterone-only pills, but irregular menses or "break-through" bleeding in mid-cycle are common and unwanted symptoms with this type of oral contraception.

The landscape of the body can be plotted using a technique called contour mapping. This method can show the subtle bodily changes that occur in early pregnancy, and during the menstrual cycle.

Couples throughout the world are becoming increasingly aware of the necessity for family planning. Different types of birth control available include hormonal, barrier and rhythm methods.

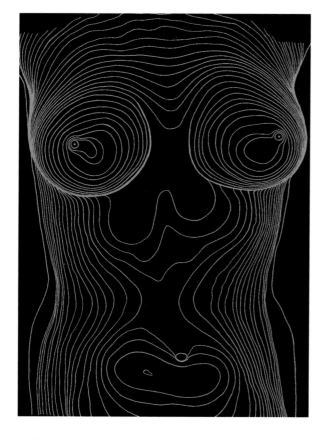

Other forms of steroid contraceptive include so-called "injectables" — injectable forms of contraceptives which usually contain progesterone only. Small deposits of this steroid are injected under the skin and released slowly from there into the bloodstream over a period of several weeks. When they were first introduced, family-planning services thought they would be ideal for contraceptives for the Third World communities who could then avoid the daily pill-taking routine. There is now some doubt about the long-term effects of these injectables, however; in fact, their use has been banned in many countries. They may in time be replaced by progesterone-releasing vaginal rings if these prove to be safe.

One major problem in testing the safety of steroid contraceptives, though, is that ideally a clinical trial should last 15 or 20 years so that the very long-term effects of the steroids can be thoroughly tested. This is not really practical.

A medication-free, but highly unreliable, method

of contraception — the rhythm method — relies on charting the hormonally controlled fluctuations in body temperature. These measurements are used to determine the points in the menstrual cycle when a woman is more unlikely to conceive, based on the fact that temperature rises slightly immediately before ovulation.

Conception and the Hormones of Pregnancy

At the mid-cycle the ripe egg bursts out of the ovary and is wafted into the Fallopian tube by whiplash movements of cilia at the open head of the tube. The egg waits for sperm penetration, but fertilization occurs only if intercourse takes place within two or three days on either side of ovulation. Sperm survive in the female reproductive tract for about 72 hours, and there is similarly only a short period when the cervical mucus is favorable for the sperm to "swim" up into the uterus and through into the Fallopian tubes.

All conditions being right, a single sperm penetrates the egg in the Fallopian tube, the two sets of chromosomes join — and fertilization has occurred. Within 24 hours the first cellular division is underway and an embryo is formed. The embryo now faces a hazardous few days, traveling down into the uterus and eventually embedding itself into the uterine lining. It takes about three to four days after fertilization for the embryo to reach the womb, at which stage it is just a little bundle of between 32 and 64 cells. Then for another three to six days it rests in the uterus, becoming a little bigger, before it "invades" the uterine lining and becomes entirely embedded in it. Meanwhile the uterus has been prepared for such an invasion through the action of estrogen and progesterone.

Pregnancy cannot be maintained, however, unless there is a continual supply of estrogen and progesterone. In the first few weeks of pregnancy these steroids come from the corpus luteum formed from the ruptured follicle after ovulation.

In all normal menstrual cycles a corpus luteum forms but breaks down (luteolysis) toward the end of the cycle; the breakdown does not take place if conception has occurred because the newly forming placenta releases a hormone very similar to luteinizing hormone. The hormone is called chorionic gonadotropin, and it maintains stimula-

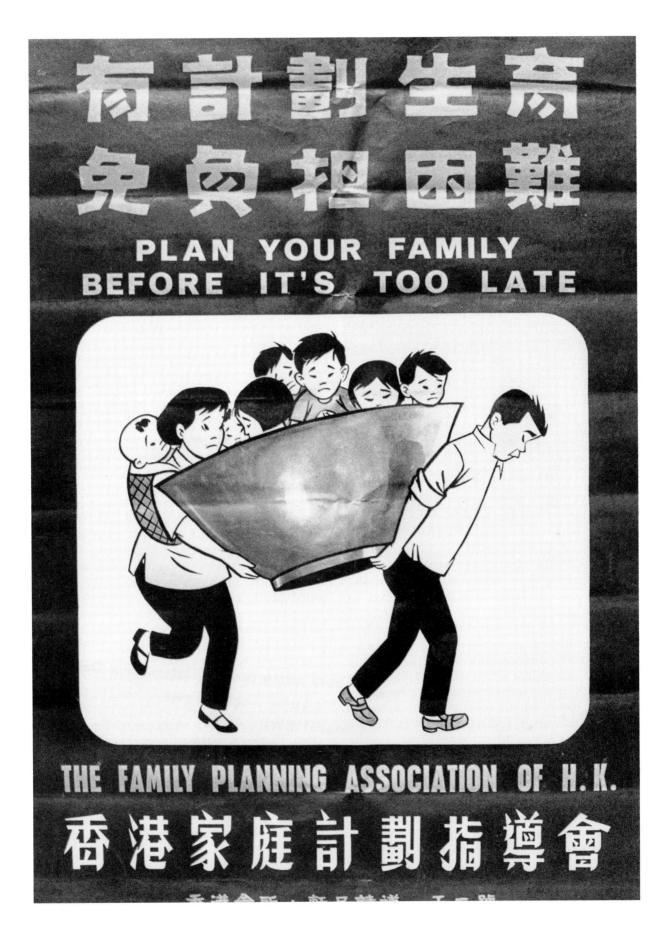

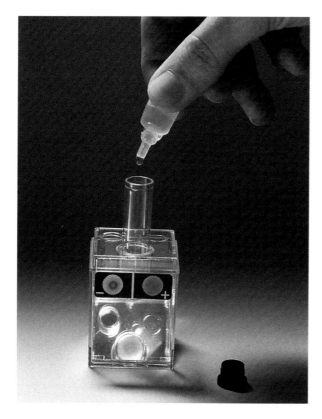

tion of the corpus luteum, so preventing luteolysis and continuing the production of estrogen and progesterone. (In fact, it is the detection of chorionic gonadotropin in the blood or urine of pregnant women that forms the basis of modern pregnancy testing.)

As the embryo burrows into the uterus it forms a placenta, an interface across which vital nutrients and oxygen can pass from the mother's blood into the fetal blood. In the reverse direction, waste products and carbon dioxide can pass from the fetal circulation back into the maternal blood. But the placenta has another important function in pregnancy: it synthesizes steroids — and after the first month of pregnancy, nearly all the steroid secretions are produced by the placenta.

The placenta takes over from the corpus luteum, although it needs the cooperations of the fetus to provide the essential estrogens. So there is a shunting of steroid hormones between the placenta and the fetus, and together they form a single endocrine organ known as the fetoplacental unit.

The placenta makes progesterone but cannot convert the progesterones to androgens. This step takes place in the liver and adrenal glands of the fetus. Then these weak androgens, with little biological activity, go back to the placenta where they are converted to estrogens.

While the fetoplacental unit busily makes these hormones, they are not directly needed by the fetus itself but by the mother. Throughout the nine months of pregnancy the levels of estrogens and progesterone in the maternal blood rise continually and bring about changes in maternal physiology that are necessary to provide the extra blood flow to the placenta and to maintain adequate nourishment for the growing baby. The mother's breasts develop, her blood volume increases, more red blood cells are needed, and more blood must be pumped through the body. There is, however, one primary action of progesterone on the uterus itself: it keeps the outer layer of muscles relaxed so that contractions of the womb are inhibited and the fetus is not expelled prematurely.

One other hormone that the placenta manufactures is placental lactogen (otherwise called somatomammotropin), which has effects similar to those of growth hormone and prolactin. It acts on the mother and alters her metabolism in a way that helps to maintain nutrients such as calcium in her blood: these nutrients are available thus to cross the placenta and provide for the baby. Most endocrinologists now agree that this placental lactogen may act as a sort of backup mechanism so that the requirements of the fetus are supplied, but how this might be the case is uncertain.

The flow of hormones between the fetus and mother through the placenta means that hormones in the fetal blood may affect the mother, and vice versa. There is an old tale that pregnant women can tell the sex of their child because they themselves become masculinized if they are carrying a boy. Certainly the testosterone released by fetal testes can get across the placenta to the mother and could produce slight signs of masculinization (such as increased hair growth on the upper lip). But equally, the lack of any masculinizing effects does not imply that the baby is a girl!

Great care must be taken not to disturb the delicate hormone balance of the mother; any

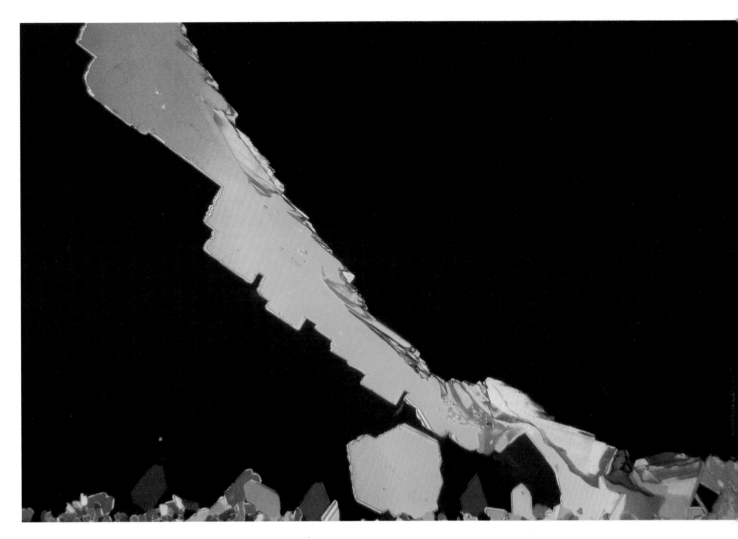

change could also alter the development of the fetus. If for example, androgens and (to a lesser extent) progestogens are given to the mother during the first three months of pregnancy, masculinization of a female fetus can result. Estrogen administration can also have serious effects. Through the late 1950s a synthetic estrogenic drug, diethylstilbestrol (DES), was given to diabetic patients to improve the prognosis of their pregnancies because the mortality among infants of diabetic mothers is greater than among normal mothers. Unfortunately, this treatment had no beneficial effect on the outcome of pregnancy, and moreover it later became apparent that the daughters of mothers who had been treated with stilbestrol were highly susceptible after adolescence to carcinoma (cancer) of the vagina.

Hormones and Childbirth

Babies are ordinarily born about 38 weeks after conception, or 40 weeks after the last menstruation, and it is remarkable that after such a long gestation

Progesterone, shown here crystallized, is a versatile hormone secreted by the female reproductive system. With other hormones, it controls the menstrual cycle and also regulates processes necessary for pregnancy, such as the preparation of the endometrium for a fertilized ovum, should conception take place.

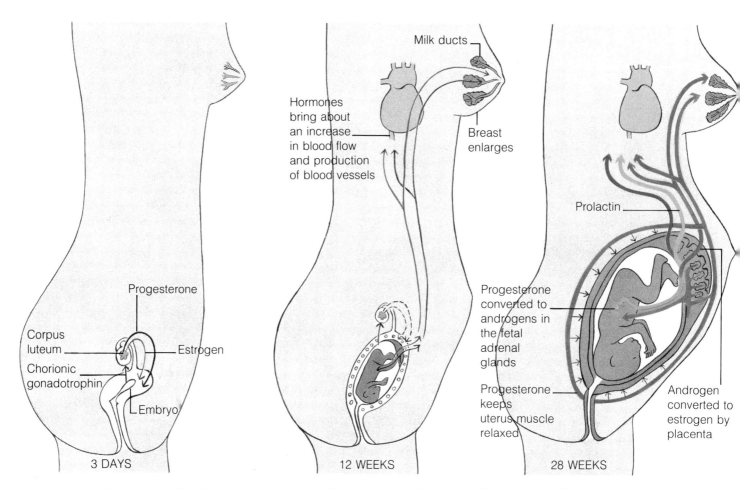

Milk ducts

Hormones bring about an increase in blood flow and production of blood vessels

Breast enlarges

Prolactin

Progesterone

Corpus luteum

Chorionic gonadotrophin

Estrogen

Embryo

Progesterone converted to androgens in the fetal adrenal glands

Progesterone keeps uterus muscle relaxed

Androgen converted to estrogen by placenta

3 DAYS   12 WEEKS   28 WEEKS

period the timing of birth is as precise as it is. It is still not absolutely known just what decides when a baby should be born. It is certainly not a simple matter of the size of the baby, because birthweight after a normal gestation period can vary from about five pounds to ten pounds. Even doubling the weight, therefore, apparently has no effect on the timing of birth.

Until fairly recently it was thought that the release of the hormone oxytocin from the posterior pituitary gland started off the contractions of the uterus which eventually push out first the baby and then the placenta. The hormone is certainly secreted during labor, but it seems to play more of a supportive role in maintaining the contractions rather than one of initiating the whole process.

Why *does* a mother go into labor? Research suggests that it is actually the baby who times his or her own birth, and that the timing is dependent on the maturation and hormone secretions of the endocrine glands — in particular the adrenal glands perched on top of each kidney. During the last few weeks of pregnancy the fetal adrenals seem to manufacture increasing amounts of androgens from progesterone. These androgens can pass back

to the placenta and be converted into estrogens. In this way the adrenal "activation" of the baby upsets the delicate hormone balance of estrogen and progesterone in the mother. The uterus no longer remains quiescent but is free to contract, and prostaglandins, along with oxytocin, stimulate the muscles of the uterus. While the contractions of labor increase in intensity and duration, the cervix softens and dilates so that when the first stage of labor is completed the cervix is perhaps about four inches in diameter.

In "natural" childbirth the baby is pushed out through the pelvis in the second stage of labor; in the third stage the placenta is delivered. For first-time mothers labor may last for about 14 hours, but in subsequent pregnancies labor is usually shorter and easier.

Right up until the moment of birth the fetus has led a sort of parasitic existence on the mother. Through the placenta the fetal blood obtains oxygen and nutrients from the maternal blood and at the same time dumps its own waste products. But after birth the baby's lungs must expand and he or she must begin to breathe. At the same time the special circulatory shunts which had enabled the

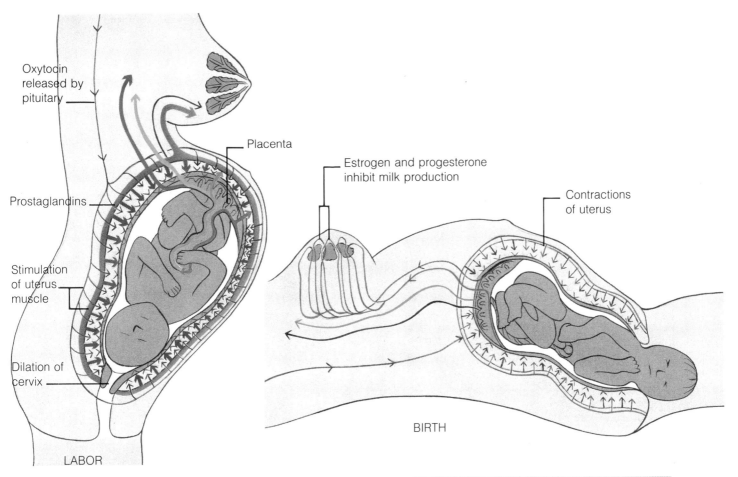

Oxytocin released by pituitary

Placenta

Prostaglandins

Stimulation of uterus muscle

Dilation of cervix

LABOR

Estrogen and progesterone inhibit milk production

Contractions of uterus

BIRTH

As soon as an egg is fertilized, the corpus luteum begins to secrete estrogen and progesterone to maintain the pregnancy. In turn, the embryo produces chorionic gonadotropin. After about twelve weeks, the corpus luteum becomes redundant when the embryo forms a placenta. Progesterone from the placenta is converted in the fetus into androgens, which are returned to the placenta to be converted into estrogen. A few weeks before birth, there is a rise in fetal androgen production. This eventually upsets the balance of estrogen and progesterone in the mother, which causes the uterus to contract. The secretion of oxytocin maintains the contractions and the baby starts its journey into the world. For the first few weeks of life the baby may be fed on breast milk. Feeding baby (right) can be a shared experience for mother and father.

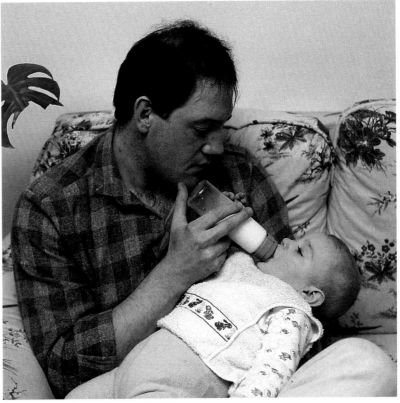

127

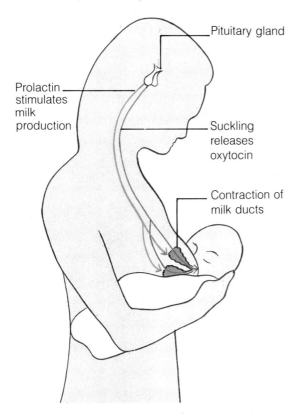

When a baby sucks at its mother's breast, the hormone oxytocin is released which causes the milk ducts to contract. In turn, this stimulates the production of prolactin, which maintains the production of milk.

Pituitary gland

Prolactin stimulates milk production

Suckling releases oxytocin

Contraction of milk ducts

fetal blood to be diverted from the lungs must shut.

The dramatic hormone changes which take place in the mother after the birth of her child enable milk production to begin. Before birth the high levels of estrogen and progesterone made by the fetoplacental unit inhibit the production of milk, even though the breasts are fully developed and prepared for lactation after the first four months of pregnancy. After delivery the levels of estrogen and progesterone fall precipitously, and prolactin is free to stimulate lactation. In the first few days a sticky fluid called colostrum is produced: it is high in proteins, vitamins and antibodies. During a transitional period lasting a week or so the concentration of proteins and antibodies in the milk decline, and after a period of between two and three weeks, mature milk is formed which has a relatively high fat and lactose concentration.

Each time the baby sucks, oxytocin is released from the posterior pituitary gland. This hormone causes the milk ducts to contract and milk to squirt out of the nipple, helping the baby to feed. At the same time the suckling stimulates secretion of the hormone prolactin which is responsible for maintaining the supply of milk. It is therefore essential that babies are suckled at frequent intervals so that prolactin is stimulated and lactation continues. This is one reason it is usually difficult for mothers to partly breast-feed and partly bottle-feed for any length of time.

Hormones and Aging in Women

The story of hormones, sexual development and fertility would not be complete without considering what happens in later life when there is progressive failure of the reproductive system. This is a phenomenon more visible in women than in men, and finally culminates for them in the menopause at around the age of forty-five to fifty-five years.

In the ten or so years preceeding the menopause (although it can be as long as twenty years), the ovaries become increasingly insensitive to the gonadotropin hormone signals. And although there are still about 10,000 immature follicles left in the ovary they fail to mature. There can thus be a prolonged period before the menopause when eggs do not ripen, the ovaries sluggishly produce hormones, and menstrual cycles are prolonged or irregular. This period is known as the climacteric. Finally, the ovaries become devoid of follicles and completely unresponsive; they are no longer capable of producing estrogens. The menopause results in a relative or absolute deficiency of steroid sex hormones.

During the climacteric and after the menopause a number of bodily and behavioral changes occur. Often it is difficult to decide whether these are caused by the estrogen withdrawal or simply by aging. Hot flashes and night sweats are common complaints of the climacteric, and post-menopausal women have an increased risk of coronary thrombosis. The uterus and glandular tissue of the breasts shrink through a lack of estrogen "support," and the secretions of the vagina change. This commonly reduces the protective mechanisms in the vagina against foreign microorganisms, and vaginitis may become a frequent problem. The loss of vaginal secretions may also cause some difficulties in intercourse which can inhibit sexual desire.

Estrogen affects bone turnover and calcium

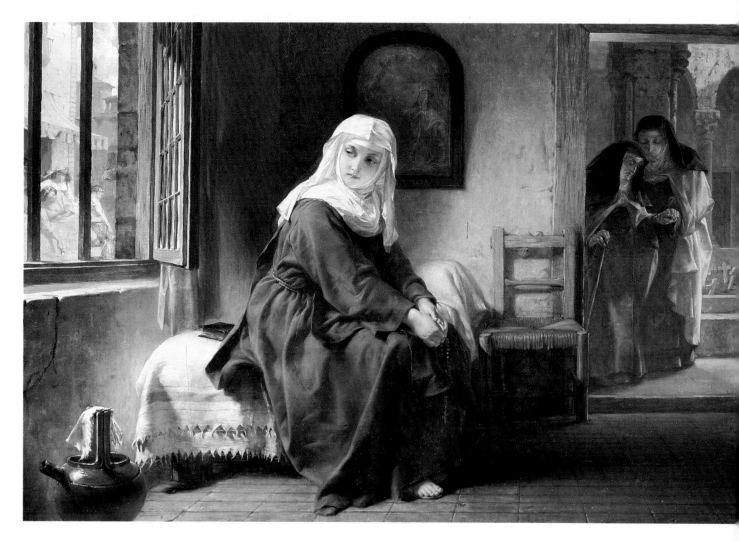

absorption from the intestine, and helps to prevent excessive breakdown or resorption of bone tissue. Lack of estrogen means that more bone is resorbed, there is a loss in total bone mass (osteoporosis), and the bones become weak and are more easily broken. Anxiety, depression and nervous tension often accompany this reproductive failure, but it is unlikely that hormonal factors are totally to blame because this is yet another period in life when a woman undergoes great psychological adjustment.

About 95 per cent of twentieth-century Western women spend approximately one-third of their lifetime in a state of estrogen deficiency. It is estimated that today as many as 30 per cent of women during this post-reproductive period warrant some form of therapy. Most commonly used is estrogen replacement therapy to alleviate symptoms of estrogen withdrawal, while behavioral counselling and psychoactive drugs are also used, singly or in combination. Estrogen replacement has also been used to slow down calcium loss from bone, with the intention of preventing fractures.

Loss of suppleness of the skin is one characteristic that takes place as part of the natural process of aging. In women this is often caused by the cessation of estrogen production during the menopause. Two centuries ago fewer than 30 per cent of women experienced such symptoms: the rest died at an earlier age.

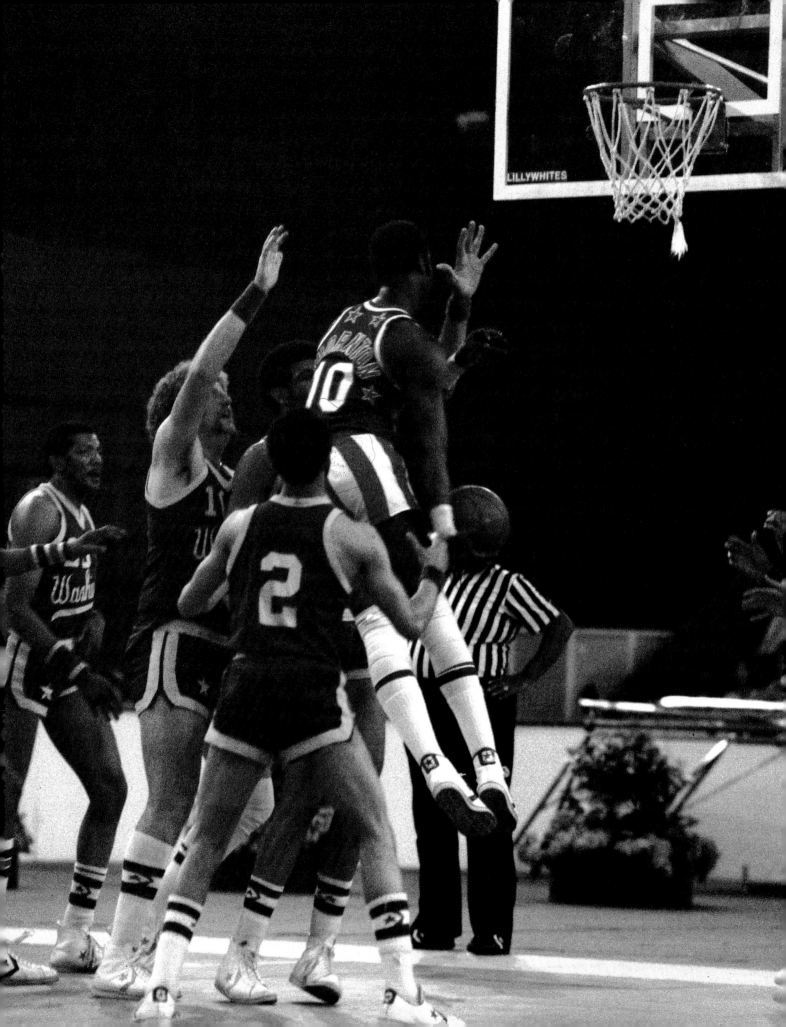

Chapter 7

Fiction or Future?

In Europe in the eighteenth century, more than 50 million people died from one disease alone; in England seventy-five per cent of the people in some towns caught a disfiguring and terrifying sickness, and because there was no cure it was accepted that chance was the only controlling factor. Smallpox is no longer left to chance, medical intervention has virtually wiped it from the face of the earth. Many other diseases have been similarly controlled and plague, diphtheria and polio are no longer accepted as major risks anywhere in the Western world.

In cases such as these there is no doubt that if terrible suffering can be prevented, then it should be. But the moral issue becomes less easy when considering the future of hormone manipulation and genetic engineering. Why should children's intelligence be left to chance when a little genetic engineering may guarantee an IQ of 150? And if stupid human beings were phased out, would the quality of our life improve? The answer to the latter question is that probably the quality of life would improve no more than social inequalities improved when smallpox was eventually eradicated.

But more optimistically, the prospects for the future uses of hormones, and the effect they are likely to have on the suffering caused by certain disorders, are increasingly encouraging.

Help for Diabetes

Diabetes mellitus is a common disorder usually caused by a deficiency or total inability of the pancreas to produce the hormone insulin. There are two forms of diabetes: insulin-independent and insulin-dependent. Insulin-independent diabetes chiefly affects persons more than 40 years old. The pancreas produces some insulin, but the body tissues such as the liver and muscles are unable to respond to it. For this form of the disorder treatment often comprises only a change of diet. Insulin-dependent, or juvenile, diabetes, usually

In possession of the ball, a Harlem Globetrotter leaps effortlessly in front of Washington Generals' defenders for a throw at the basket. The sheer height of these players, many of whom are more than seven feet tall, contributes greatly to their amazing agility and skill. If a combination of genetic heritage, nutrition and other environmental considerations can produce exceptionally tall individuals, it is interesting to speculate whether or not it might eventually be possible to program an individual's height by manipulating the gene responsible for growth hormone production.

131

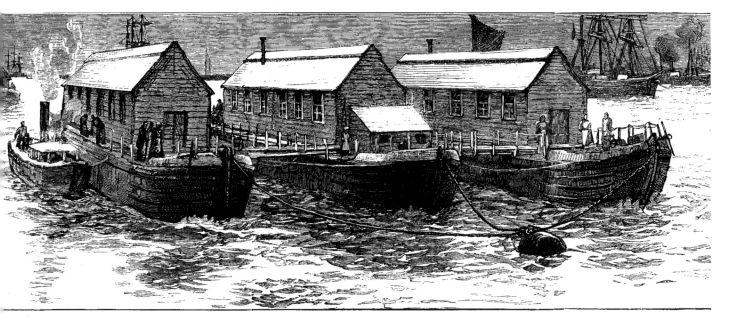

occurs in young people and is characterized by the failure of the pancreas to produce insulin.

Symptoms of insulin-dependent diabetes can be prevented by regular doses of insulin, and at present these come from two sources: animal and human. Animal insulin is comparatively easy to get from slaughtered cattle or hogs — but unfortunately some patients become allergic to it. They need the other source, human insulin, and until recently obtaining the hormone was a costly process. Human insulin can be removed from the pancreas during autopsy, but this is completely impractical because the pancreas begins to degenerate from the moment of death. And it would not be possible to get enough insulin from this source to treat all the diabetics who needed it.

Human insulin can be taken from blood plasma, but this is also fraught with difficulties. Only very small quantities can be purified from human blood plasma given by donors, and recently the presence of infectious agents such as hepatitis B and AIDS virus has made the collection and processing of human blood more complex, thus further restricting supplies.

Now a solution has emerged. It is possible to make available large quantities of pure human hormones using the biochemical technique of genetic engineering. The problem that faced the

engineer was to get cells to produce hormones outside the natural environment of the body.

The functioning of the hormone-producing cell is the key to understanding how genetic engineering works. A cell consists of a nucleus surrounded by cytoplasm. The nucleus of every cell contains strands of DNA, making up the chromosomes which carry an organism's inherited genetic information — the genes.

The genes of each cell possess a library of instructions for every function of every cell in the body. A cell that is programmed to produce insulin, for example, passes the request to do so to the nucleus, where the insulin gene in turn instructs organelles in the cytoplasm to begin production of the hormone. If the same cell receives an instruction to produce thyroid hormone it refuses to do so, because it is programmed to accept only commands to produce insulin. It is possible, however, for viruses to find their way into cells where, once inside, they reproduce hundreds of times. This knowledge has been useful to the genetic engineer.

When producing insulin artificially, the engineer extracts the gene containing the insulin instructions from the library of genes held on a chromosome. It is then inserted into a minute bacterial chromosome called a plasmid. The new insulin gene must be inserted into the plasmid in exactly the right place,

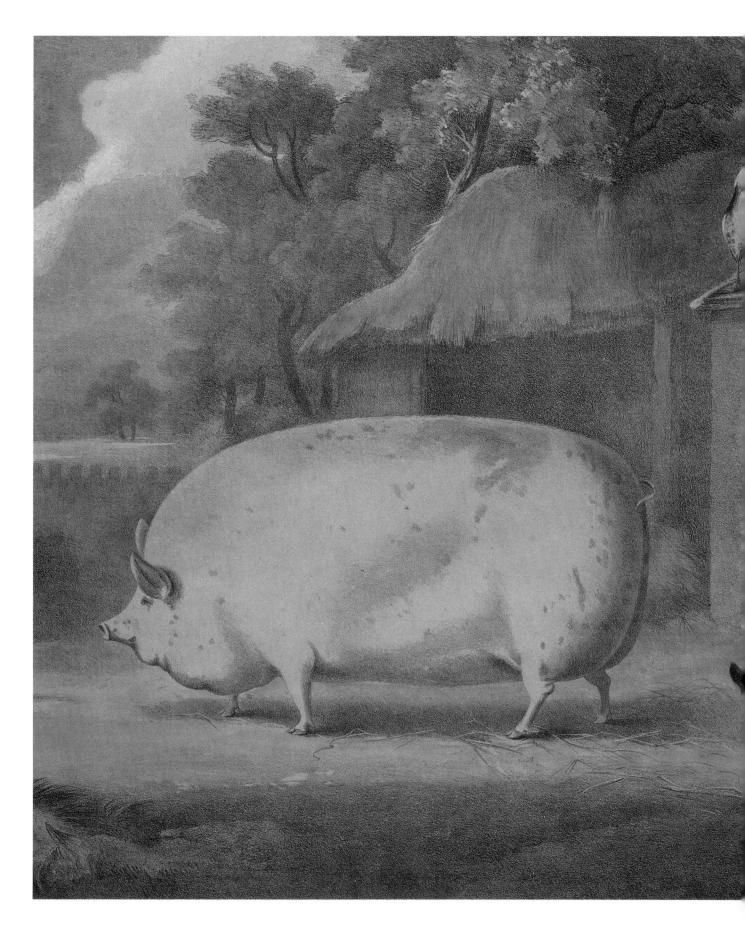

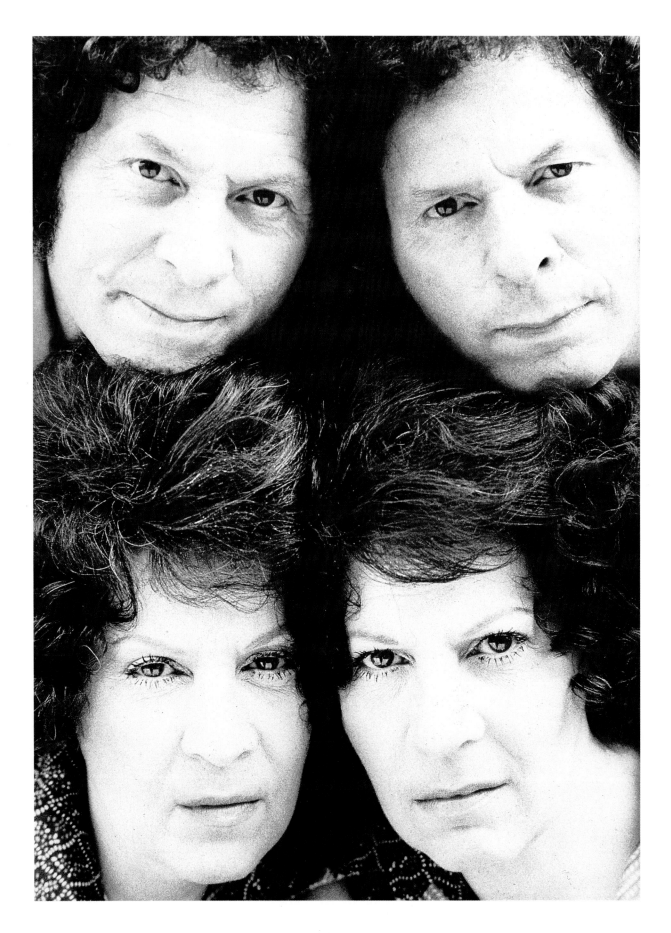

so that signals from the plasmid have the effect of
reprogramming the cell to switch to the production
of insulin. The plasmid containing the new gene is
then put back into the bacteria, which treat it as one
of their own, thus enabling the production of
insulin in large quantities.

The bacteria, with the plasmid containing the
human hormone gene, are grown in huge tanks
called fermenters which carefully control the
temperature, nutrient supply and oxygen content
to maximize production. If all of the genetic
engineering goes correctly, large quantities of the
hormone can be produced in the fermenter and be
purified for clinical investigation.

Genetic engineering has brightened the future of
treatment for diabetes. An allergic patient can be
treated without any adverse reactions and, in
addition, patients treated with human insulin from
the beginning of their illness may never develop
allergic reactions because they have always
received a protein identical to the one they lack.

Growth Hormone Manufactured

The second hormone just becoming available can
help to treat children whose growth has slowed
down because they lack growth hormone.

Most of the growth hormone available today is
produced from human pituitary glands removed
after death. The hormone is stable, but only very
small quantities can be produced, severely restricting the supply. This forces clinicians to make
difficult decisions about who should receive
treatment and who should not.

Recently three people who received growth
hormone from cadaver pituitary glands developed
a rare type of viral brain infection. The virus was
probably a contaminant of the growth hormone
preparation used. In consequence, however, the
use of pituitary-derived growth hormone has now
been banned by the Food and Drug Administration
(FDA). This makes licensing and release of
genetically-engineered growth hormone an urgent
matter since it is now the only safe and economic
source of the hormone.

The unlimited supply made possible by genetic
engineering is bound to raise a whole new set of
ethical problems. It is not fully understood why a
person stops growing when he or she reaches a

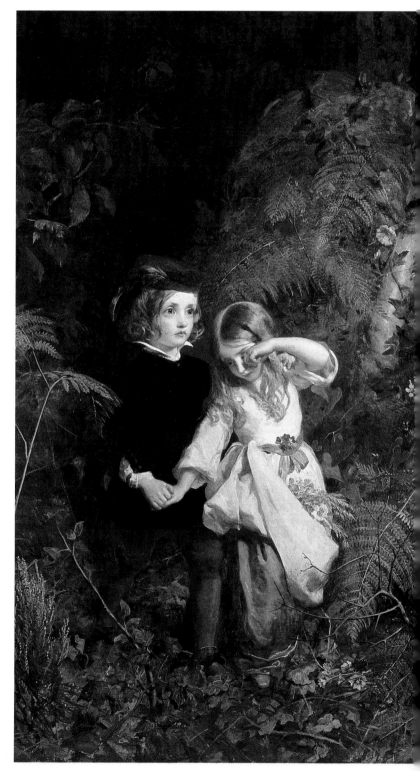

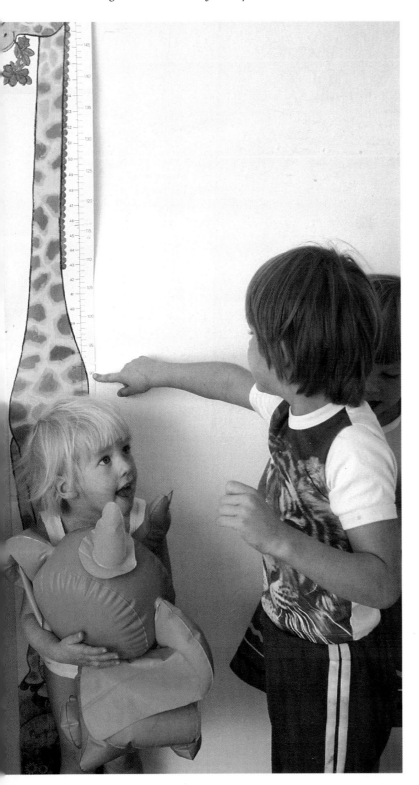

Preschool children measure how tall they have grown. There is a wide range of heights even for normal, healthy children, but if growth is retarded or accelerated, a hormonal growth disorder may be responsible.

certain height, but it is possible that growth hormone could make any child grow faster and taller than would normally be expected.

A continuous oversupply of growth hormone is known to produce the condition known as gigantism, which has many severe complications. What no one knows is the results of a short course of treatment. This could increase a child's height by a few inches, and if this was the case there could be a demand to increase the size of a normal child who was shorter than average. There may even be parents who demand treatment for their children so that they all grow to six feet tall or more. Clearly the use of growth hormone will require careful medical and ethical consideration if its use is not to become abused. There is an interesting historical parallel to this phenomenon. In Britain in the tenth century members of the aristocracy towered over the common people because they ate an adequate diet whereas most of their subjects did not. Their extra height made them physically superior.

Intellectual Enhancement

Vasopressin (antidiuretic hormone) is made in the hypothalamus and released from the posterior pituitary to help maintain fluid balance.

Recent technological advances have made supplies of the hormone both plentiful and inexpensive and have permitted investigation of some of its other properties. Because vasopressin is also found in parts of the brain aside from the hypothalamus, it was thought that it might somehow be involved in certain brain functions. Tests were carried out in which individuals were given small quantities of the hormone in a nasal spray (so that the hormone could be absorbed rapidly into the bloodstream through the nasal mucosa). These individuals were then given a number of psychological tests, which showed that the hormone could improve short-term memory. There are many implications for the future of such a drug, for both students and people suffering from memory loss associated with aging, although there are also ethical problems to be considered.

Administration of Hormones Improves

When adequate quantities of hormones are available for all who need them, the next most pressing

Robert Merrifield

The Science of Synthesis

Robert Merrifield is presently Professor of Biochemistry at Rockefeller University in New York. That he works and teaches at a Rockefeller establishment is entirely appropriate, for it was at the Rockefeller Institute in 1930 that John Northrop first crystallized pepsin and showed that it was a protein. And Professor Merrifield is famous in turn for his development of solid-phase peptide synthesis, and for being the first scientist to synthesize an enzyme.

Merrifield was born at Fort Worth, Texas, in July 1921. He graduated at the University of California at Los Angeles (UCLA) in 1943 and attained a doctorate there six years later. His first post was as chemist at the Philip R. Park Research Foundation, but by the time his doctorate came through he was already assistant chemist at UCLA, from where he progressed through various positions to become Associate Professor in 1966. In that year he left to take up his present post. Concurrently he is associate editor of the *International Journal of Peptide and Protein Research*, a function he has performed successfully since 1969.

Ingested proteins break down to smaller degraded units—the peptides, which are then absorbed through the

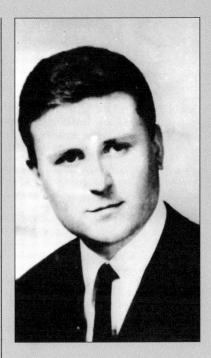

stomach or intestine into the bloodstream or broken down further by pancreatic enzymes. The peptides, then, are our main source of energy. Synthesis of them is thus both a practical and useful notion. And it is in synthesizing peptides that Merrifield's talent has been conspicuous. In particular, it was he who managed to find a relationship between the structure and the function of synthetic biologically-active peptides and proteins.

His original method of peptide synthesis was to devise a process by which a peptide molecule was attached to a

polymer "bead" so that during a sequence of additions of individual amino acids (separated each time by a process of washing), a carefully constructed peptide chain could gradually be pieced together. The method has proved reasonably effective, especially in the synthesis of the less complex peptides, although it was quickly found that the polymer bead tended to deteriorate through all the successive washings, and an inorganic substitute (a silica gel or controlled pore glass) is presently preferred.

Merrifield's work has resulted in considerable further research into the uses and the synthesis of peptides. One—aspartame—has been used as a noncalorific sweetener in some US soft drinks. But, possibly more valuably, scientists at the Scripps Clinic at La Jolla, California, in 1983 synthesized a peptide that "mimics" small regions of a virus's outer coating so successfully that it causes the formation in a human of antibodies capable of neutralizing that virus, and can thus be used as a vaccine in immune programs.

Professor Merrifield has won several international awards for his pioneering research, including the Nobel Prize in 1985.

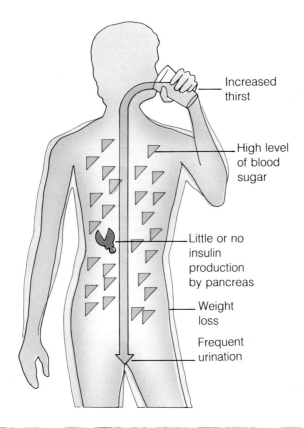

Increased thirst

High level of blood sugar

Little or no insulin production by pancreas

Weight loss

Frequent urination

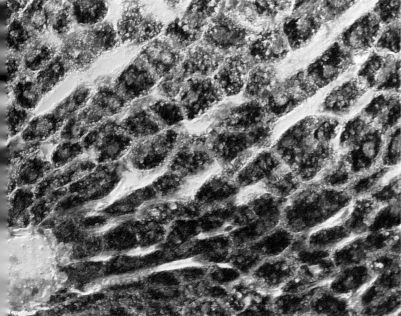

problem is to find the best way to administer them. The interrelationship between hormones and metabolic products is complex indeed; for example, a rise in blood sugar after a meal is followed by a rapid rise in insulin secretion which in turn makes the blood sugar level fall again. It is impossible to mimic this sort of rapid cyclical response by injections of insulin, which are usually widely spaced during the day for the convenience of the patient and to stop blood sugar levels from becoming too high or too low.

An ideal solution would be to couple a sensitive detector of sugar levels to a continuous source of insulin, then the hormone could be supplied when blood sugar rises, but could be shut off rapidly when sugar levels fall. This sort of pumping device might be able to keep sugar levels "normal" throughout the day and night, monitoring and responding to tiny fluctuations, and the improved standard of control would potentially prevent many of the complications of this common disorder (such as kidney disease and blindness).

Prototypes of such pumps are being tried out, but at present they have to be strapped to the body and connected to fine tubes implanted under the skin. The pumps deliver insulin only according to a pre-set program. Machines which first measure glucose

The main symptoms of diabetes mellitus (above) occur as a result of excess glucose in the blood. The excess "overflows" into the urine, causing an increase in the frequency of urination. This loss of fluid makes an untreated diabetic perpetually thirsty. Glucose-starvation of the body's cells can cause tiredness and weight-loss because fat and muscle are burned up to provide energy. Regular urine or blood tests are used to check blood glucose levels. If blood glucose is too high, it can be reduced by taking insulin, which aids in transporting glucose from the blood for storage in muscle and liver tissues (left). These tissues release glucose into the blood when the body needs energy.

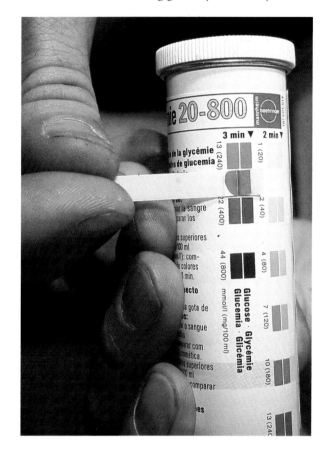

To measure blood glucose levels, a diabetes test-strip is first soaked in a small sample of blood, and the resulting color change compared with a chart. This one shows a high level: 280 mg glucose per 100 ml of blood.

levels before delivering the required amount of insulin are presently too large to be worn by a patient. The ultimate device would be one that a patient could have implanted under the skin like a heart pacemaker—a type already on the horizon.

Considerable research is being carried out on different ways to administer insulin to diabetics. For example, it is now possible to modify a human insulin gene in such a way that all its properties stay the same except for one. It is no longer susceptible to attack by acid and digestive enzymes. Given this ability a diabetic would be able to take the hormone by mouth rather than by injection. Another area of research is into the manufacture of a "liver-seeking" variant that could be taken up by liver cells in preference to other cells in the body. An additional approach is the administration of insulin by nasal spray to avoid multiple injections.

In a healthy person the insulin from the pancreas travels to the liver through the veins that carry blood from the intestines. Endocrinologists believe that complications of the disease could be further lessened if this natural transportation were mimicked. Were it not for the high risk of infection, this could be done by injecting insulin directly into the blood vessels of the abdomen. Instead it has been suggested that a piece of the intra-abdominal tissue called the omentum could be moved from the abdomen to a new site, just beneath the skin, so that an injection into these veins would deliver the insulin directly where it is needed in the liver.

The Perfect Solution

Although diabetes can be controlled, how much more satisfactory it would be if the islets that have ceased insulin production could be replaced.

Unfortunately the normal pancreas is difficult to transplant because it has a complex blood supply and is liable to "self-destruct" because of its large content of digestive enzymes. To overcome this problem, attempts have been made to transplant isolated islets or islet cells to diabetics. This is done by injecting islets into the portal veins running to the liver, where they are bathed in normal nutrients from the gastrointestinal tract. This system is still unreliable, however, because the body responds to the new islet cells as foreign material. The natural immune system is stimulated and the cells are

rejected. Potentially with more effective immuno-suppressive drugs and as surgical techniques continue to improve, this permanent and ideal answer to diabetes may become possible.

Prevention—Better than Cure

The mystery of diabetes is gradually being unraveled. It is known, for example, that diabetic children have a particular antibody (called an anti-islet cell antibody) which reacts with the islet cells in their pancreases. This antibody is often found in the blood at the time that the disorder first becomes apparent. The antibody is not in itself the cause of diabetes, but it is detectable in some children before there are any clinical signs of the disorder, which suggests that diabetic symptoms follow a long period of gradual islet cell destruction rather than a single catastrophic event.

In the light of this information, attempts are now being made to detect potentially diabetic children

Food digested in the intestine releases glucose into the blood. In a healthy person, this increase in blood sugar level causes the islets of Langerhans in the pancreas to release insulin. The increased secretion of insulin maintains blood sugar at a steady level by accelerating the passage of glucose into insulin receptive tissues, such as the liver or muscles. In a diabetic individual, the pancreas fails to produce insulin when stimulated by glucose. To prevent a build-up of glucose, insulin is introduced artificially. In a matter of seconds the insulin enters the blood, where it transports the glucose to the receptive organs.

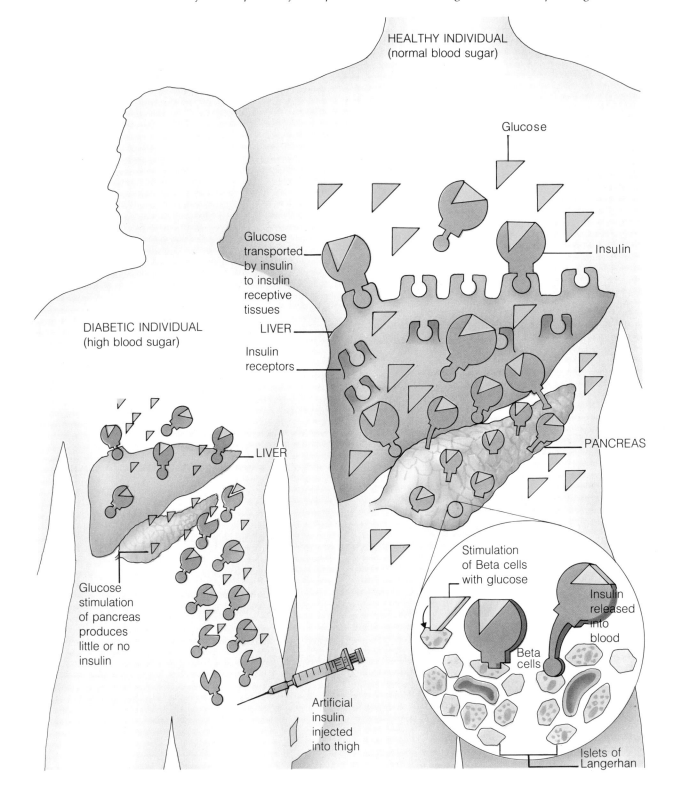

HEALTHY INDIVIDUAL
(normal blood sugar)

Glucose

Glucose transported by insulin to insulin receptive tissues

Insulin

DIABETIC INDIVIDUAL
(high blood sugar)

LIVER

Insulin receptors

LIVER

PANCREAS

Glucose stimulation of pancreas produces little or no insulin

Stimulation of Beta cells with glucose

Insulin released into blood

Beta cells

Artificial insulin injected into thigh

Islets of Langerhan

before they develop any symptoms of the disease. This can be done in some families in which one child has already developed the disorder, indicating that the siblings are at a higher risk than the average. Tissue markers very similar to blood groups can help identify siblings at special risk.

Once these children have been identified it may be possible to halt the progressive loss of insulin-secreting cells by early treatment with immuno-suppressive drugs such as cyclosporin A. However, at present no one knows exactly how likely these "high risk" children are to develop diabetes, so early intervention may not be wholly justified. Children may receive at best unnecessary, and at worst potentially harmful, treatment for a disorder they may never develop.

A better compromise seems to be intervention just as the symptoms begin. Because the disease is caused by gradual loss, a patient may develop symptoms of insulin deficiency before he or she has lost all of the insulin-secreting cells. Some patients develop a temporary remission of symptoms for a few weeks or months, during which insulin secretion returns before it finally disappears forever. Immunosuppressive treatment might prevent further damage and salvage some residual islet-cell function, and the need for a lifetime of insulin injections could be prevented. Trials of this type of therapy are already in progress even though it is too soon to say how beneficial the system will prove to be.

Why a person's body should reject islet cells remains a mystery, but two theories have been suggested. One is that diabetes is an autoimmune disease and that in some people the body's white blood cells (lymphocytes) attack the islet cells. If this is the case, then immunosuppressive therapy probably provides the best option. But there is some evidence that virus infections may be responsible for islet cell damage in at least some cases; as yet, no single virus has been implicated.

It is more likely that diabetes is an uncommon complication that can occur after several different virus infections. If this is the case, the identification of even a few viruses might make it possible to develop vaccines against them to prevent infection by the dangerous agent. The future may witness the introduction of a cocktail vaccine, which would

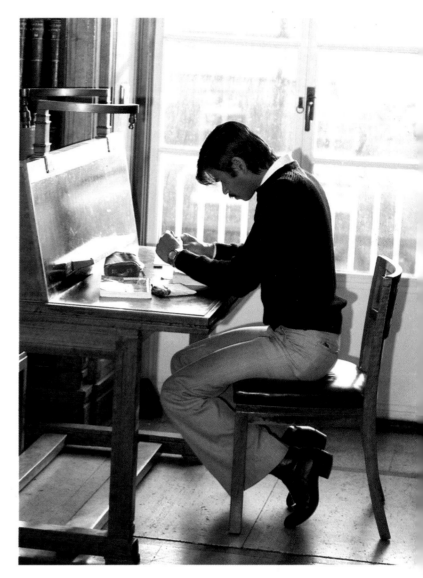

Last-minute cramming before an examination can sometimes work wonders. Key points fresh in the memory can suddenly come flooding back just at that all-important moment. Unfortunately we can hold only a limited amount of information in short-term memory. Recent developments in medical technology have isolated the hormone vasopressin from the brain and shown that it can produce enhancement of short-term memory.

Javelin throwers are among athletes who theoretically could benefit from taking anabolic steroids to improve strength and endurance. Steroids have, however, been found to cause harmful effects such as liver damage.

Peak performance in a gymnast, requiring suppleness and body control, can be adversely affected by physical changes at puberty. This may have tempted some to take medication to delay puberty.

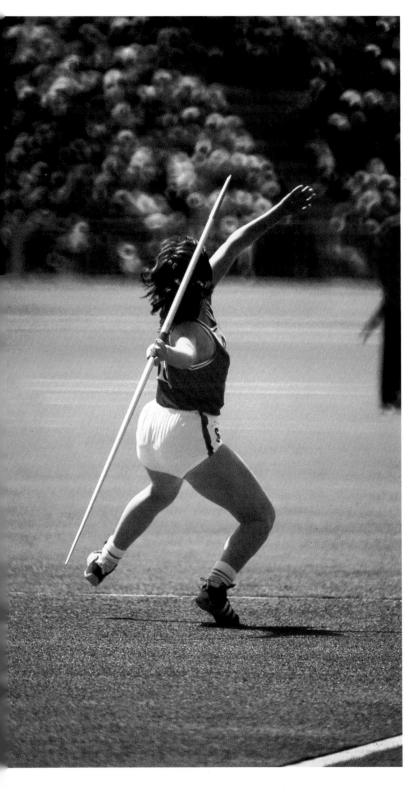

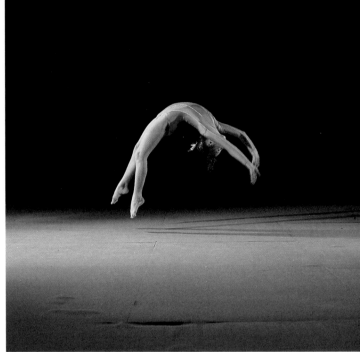

consist of a mixture capable of preventing infection by any one of several different viruses.

Steroid Hormones

Naturally produced steroid hormones have many and varied effects on the body, but their deliberate use in sport as "body modifiers" causes much controversy. The taking of anabolic steroids is banned in most sports but these substances are still used illegally by specialists in strength events such as shot-put and hammer-throwing. The male sex hormone testosterone is an anabolic steroid which (with its chemical relatives) increases muscle size. It is now clear that the muscle fibers themselves do not increase in number or size, but that the salt and water content within the fibers increases. Why this should improve performance is uncertain, but one suggestion is that anabolic steroids increase the individual's capacity for training by allowing more exercise for longer periods of time. Thus the athlete is fitter and can stress his or her body harder. Another theory is based on the fact that steroid hormones can sometimes have dramatic effects on personality when used in clinical medicine.

Perhaps the anabolic steroids interact with other natural hormones to increase the desire to train and speed up recovery from fatigue.

The cynical comment that modern sport is often a competition between two pharmacologists rather than two athletes may sometimes be true. For example, a number of chemicals similar to testosterone are under surreptitious development for use in sport. The aim is to produce compounds that have the same performance-enhancing effects as testosterone, but which cannot be detected by the dope tests performed under the auspices of international sporting bodies.

Anabolic steroids are not merely wonder-drugs prohibited to make the game fairer. Taking them can be dangerous, because they raise a person's blood pressure by increasing salt and water retention. Some preparations may inhibit sperm production in men and lead to infertility. Many of these side effects are not restricted to the time the athlete uses the drug but may be long-term. For example, there is an increase in the incidence of both benign and malignant liver tumors. In addition, arterial disease may be aggravated by the drug. In some sports, such as weight lifting, it is possible to boost the power of muscles beyond the strength of the bones and joints to which they are attached. This can lead to catastrophic joint damage caused by a sudden rupture of ligaments and tendons. The consequences of some damage may not become apparent until later, when an athlete may find himself crippled by osteoarthritis caused by damage to the cartilage on the surface of a joint.

Modifying Natural Hormones

International panels testing for hormone use have an added problem to simple drug administration, and that is to determine whether athletes have been involved in techniques that modify normal hormone responses. This is particularly common among some sportswomen, especially swimmers and gymnasts who usually "peak" before puberty. The psychological and physical changes that occur during and after puberty have devastating effects on their performance. American coaches have suspected that deliberate puberty-delaying treatment has been used in Eastern European countries. Investigations are underway to discover exactly

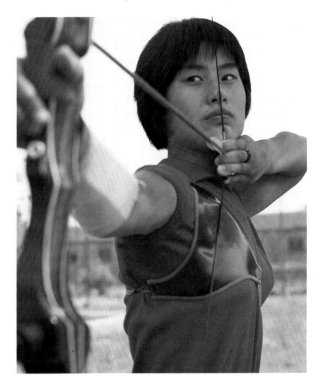

An archer has to overcome the symptoms of anxiety that can interfere with his concentration. In theory, beta-blockers could be taken to curb the symptoms by reducing pulse rate and blood pressure.

how this is done, and whether or not it should be made illegal.

A more acceptable field of exploration is in the normal hormonal cycles and their control. Everyone has a diurnal (daily) rhythm of hormonal production which varies subtly from person to person. As far as an athlete is concerned, there may be a particular time of day when the hormonal balance is optimal for training and competition. Better understanding of this natural process might make it possible to adjust an individual's inherent rhythm for a particular event.

Jet lag is a related problem caused by complex adjustments to movement across time zones. For an athlete or business person it can be disastrous if he or she is in a "hormone trough" at a time requiring peak performance. It is possible that a natural hormone such as melatonin could be given to produce a rapid normalization of the hormone cycle, allowing the athlete to perform at maximum level immediately.

So what does the future hold for the manipulation of both natural and artificial hormones? Undoubtedly such manipulation will continue, and

Diurnal rhythms play a significant part in human life, affecting metabolism, sleep and wakefulness, and mental performance. The marked cycle of hydrocortisone levels in the blood is one important hormonal rhythm. The secretion of hydrocortisone from the adrenals is stimulated by the release of adrenocorticotropic hormone (ACTH) from the pituitary. It is thought to play a part in regulating the blood levels of some white cells in the blood, sleep and consciousness, and the heart and lungs. Rhythmic fluctuations in body temperature seem to be closely related to mental performance. Body temperature is

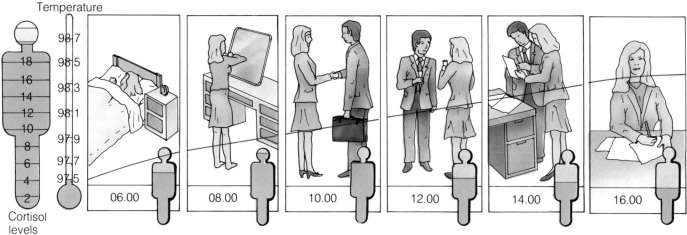

Temperature

Cortisol levels mg/100ml

06.00　08.00　10.00　12.00　14.00　16.00

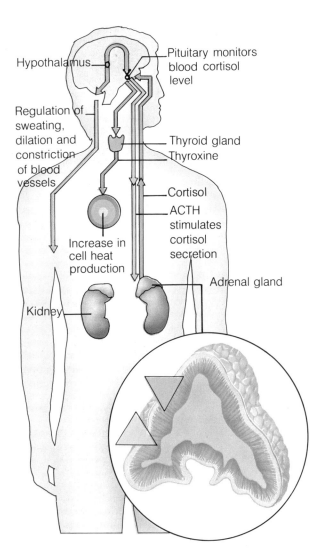

Hypothalamus

Pituitary monitors blood cortisol level

Regulation of sweating, dilation and constriction of blood vessels

Thyroid gland

Thyroxine

Cortisol

ACTH stimulates cortisol secretion

Increase in cell heat production

Adrenal gland

Kidney

as methods of detection improve, different substances will come under increasingly close scrutiny.

The problems in sport are bound to increase now that rare, expensive, natural hormones such as growth hormone are more freely available. It is reasonable to suggest that this hormone, which increases strength and stamina, should be banned along with anabolic steroids. If a sportsman has a short course of growth hormone, his performance improves—but by the time he comes up for dope testing all detectable residue is gone from his system. A ban will be difficult to enforce.

Another question is: should beta-blocker drugs be banned in sports? These drugs were developed to treat high blood pressure and coronary artery disease, and they inhibit one of the receptors in the tissues which "binds" the hormone epinephrine. In a healthy person the epinephrine produces a rapid pulse, a fine tremor (shivering or shaking sensation), a dry mouth — all symptoms of anxiety that every performer or competitor feels to a greater or lesser extent. On the other hand, for a sport such as archery or target shooting, this response is a definite hindrance. The competitor may be locked in a cycle of anxiety making him or her perform poorly. Beta-blockers inhibit pulse rate and blood pressure and enhance such a competitor's ability to concentrate.

Steroid Hormones in Treatment

Also called glucocorticoids, the steroid hormones have significant effects on many types of cancer,

144

controlled by the hypothalamus which influences the secretion of the hormone thyroxine by the thyroid gland. This is turn speeds up the rate at which cells consume oxygen, metabolize glucose and produce heat.

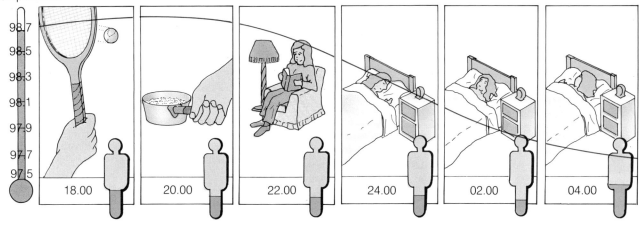

especially tumors of the breast, prostate gland and lymphoid cells. This is not surprising since these tissues are normally very responsive to steroids and have specific receptors for them in their cell cytoplasm.

An American surgeon, Charles Huggins, shared the 1966 Nobel Prize in medicine for his work showing that such tumors could be treated by hormone manipulation. At one time the only solution was to remove the hormone-producing tissue such as the adrenal glands, ovaries or testes. Now such drastic treatment is not considered necessary except in unusual circumstances. New drugs, some already in clinical use, can be used to shut off gland function. These compounds bind tightly to the same receptors as the normal hormones but block the cell's response, rather like plugging a safety cover into an electric socket. Naturally occurring hormones cannot then make the cell grow because their receptors are occupied. In the future many more antireceptor agents may become available to inhibit tumors which require normal hormones for their growth and spread.

The presence of hormone receptors in some tumors such as breast and uterine cancer give a good indication of the probable course of the illness. A patient with such receptors has a better outlook than one without, because the receptor-containing tumor is more likely to respond to receptor-blocking agents. New tests based on antibodies to specific receptors have added a new dimension to cancer therapy. It is possible to predict which patients will do well and guide the choice of drugs for chemotherapy.

Hormones Reduce Further Suffering

Locally-acting hormones (autocoids) such as the prostaglandins and their chemical cousins, the leukotrienes, seem to play a central role in tissue damage. Under intense investigation at present is their role in inflammation and their part in blood clotting and blood vessel disease.

Rheumatoid arthritis is a painful and disabling disease which is fairly common. Both aspirin and indomethacin are partly effective at controlling the inflammation associated with the condition, and it seems that the drugs inhibit the enzymes which form prostaglandins inside the cells. Unfortunately, the enzymes responsible for leukotriene formation are still produced, and there is an active search for a drug that will inhibit or block these as well. The use of synthetic relatives of this group of autocoids may bring much of the inflammatory process to a halt.

A significant interaction between two members of the prostaglandin family occurs in the walls of blood vessels. Endothelial cells make a substance called prostacyclin which inhibits blood clotting, whereas blood platelets make thromboxane which enhances clotting. In normal vessels these substances are balanced and the blood can flow freely through the veins and arteries without clotting. If an artery is diseased, however, there may be a deficiency of prostacyclin formation and the chance

*Commercial fermentation units (top)
are employed to produce large
quantities of hormones, often used in
the treatment of disease. The
hormone insulin is now produced
artificially for the treatment of*

*diabetes. In the future, research may
isolate hormones that prevent or
alleviate the symptoms of many other
disorders, including perhaps the
painful joint inflammation associated
with rheumatoid arthritis (bottom).*

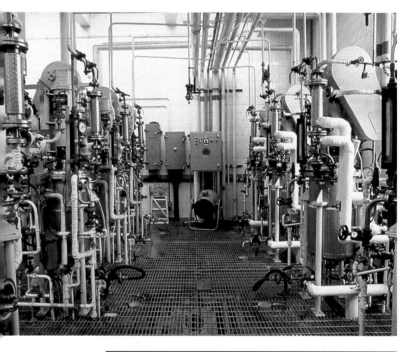

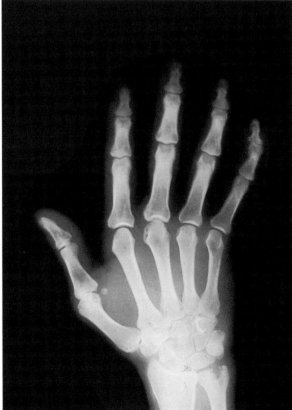

of a clot (thrombosis) forming is thus greater. This may be the reason that clots form and cause conditions such as myocardial infarction (heart attack), cerebral thrombosis (stroke) and gangrene of the legs caused by arterial thrombosis.

Experiments have begun with the first prostacyclin-like agents, and if these prove successful similar synthetic compounds could be used to treat a whole range of arterial problems.

Fertility and Contraception

Hormone manipulation has been used to control fertility for many years in the form of the contraceptive pill, but the method is not entirely satisfactory. In less-developed countries a longer-lasting agent that could be taken (or administered) once a year would be a great advantage, freeing women of the burden of having to remember to take a pill every day. Attempts are currently being made to produce a hormone in an oil base which can be injected under the skin, with the hormone gradually released into the blood supply; early field trials suggest this method is effective.

Similar research is continuing into finding an inhibitor of sperm production. There are good prospects of finding a long-acting male contraceptive. One additional advantage of this type of agent is that the effects are temporary, so that a man could regain his fertility if and when he wanted to. The system should prove less expensive than vasectomy, which not only involves surgery but is also virtually irreversible.

Another new nonsurgical method of contraceptive sounds as it if has come from the realms of science fiction — a vaccine against sperm. It is based on the observation that many prostitutes form antibodies against sperm and become conception-resistant to conceiving. Experimental evidence suggests that antisperm antibodies seem to work by inhibiting the movement of the sperm. A vaccine may still be only a distant prospect, but it would replace the need to manipulate a woman's hormonal cycle. An alternative possible vaccine would immunize a woman so that she makes antibodies to the pregnancy-sustaining hormone chorionic gonadotropin. If the antibody prevented or curtailed the action of the hormone, the pregnancy would end at a very early stage.

Charles Huggins

Pioneer in Chemotherapy

Today, one of the three major forms of treatment for cancer is chemotherapy—the use of chemical agents, particularly hormonal extracts. But such a practice only eventuated through the work of Charles Brenton Huggins in 1939 when, taking to a logical conclusion an item of information that had been common medical knowledge for some time, he arrived at an innovatory idea.

Born in Halifax, Nova Scotia, in September 1901, Huggins graduated from Acadia University, Wolfsville, but went to Harvard for his doctorate in 1924. Three years later he joined the faculty of the University of Chicago Medical School, where he remained for half a century. Between 1951 and 1969 he was also director of the May Laboratory of Cancer Research.

He became a naturalized US citizen in 1933.

Huggins' great idea came in the light of the fact that the prostate gland was known to be controlled by the male sex hormones (androgens). He therefore concluded that a tumor in the prostate might be effectively treated by isolating it from the presence of androgens (which are produced by the testes).

Following this line of thought his initial form of

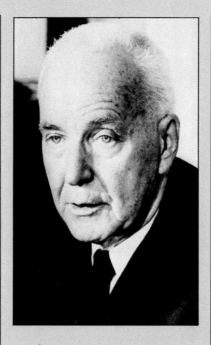

treatment on patients with prostate tumors was, to say the least, radical: castration. But in most of the patients on whom it was performed, the method proved to have some beneficial effects; in some their conditions were alleviated and in others the tumors gave no further problems at all (although in all cases there were natural and inevitable side effects).

It then occurred to Huggins that there was an alternative to radical orchiectomy; instead of eliminating androgens altogether from the body, it might be just as effective somehow to neutralize them— to administer female sex

hormones in quantity sufficient to have an identical effect on the prostate.

And so, in 1941, he began to use injections of the hormones stilbestrol and hexestrol. (Stilbestrol is still used in the form of a white, crystalline powder—diethylstilbestrol— as an estrogenic part of hormone replacement therapy for menopausal problems and to assist suppressed lactation. Hexestrol is a hydrogenated form of diethylstilbestrol.)

The treatment marked the first purely chemical medication against cancer.

Other experimenters at once tested different hormonal injections, some with success, and at least a basic form of chemotherapy was established for several types of tumor. Particularly useful was the treatment by some of Huggins' followers of women suffering from cancer in the breast. Treated with the male hormone testosterone, at least one patient in six measurably benefited.

For his work Huggins received the Nobel Prize in medicine for 1966, aged 65. In fact he shared it with Peyton Rous (then aged 85), the discoverer of the viruses which cause some cancers in animals; both scientists were awarded the Prize some time after their pioneering works.

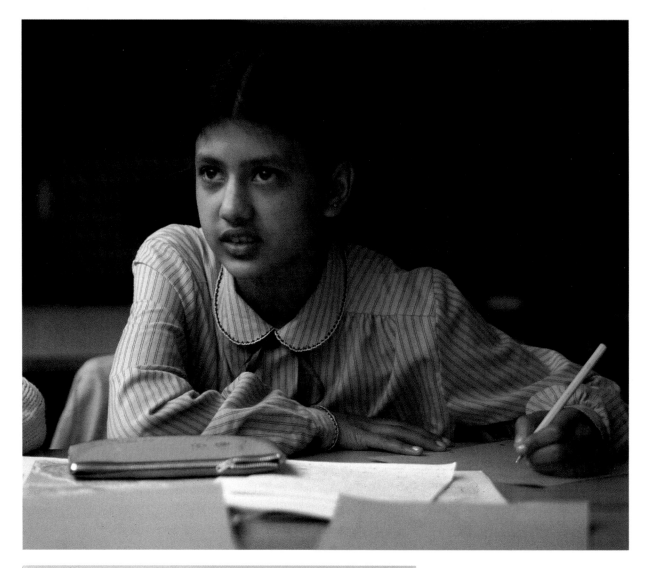

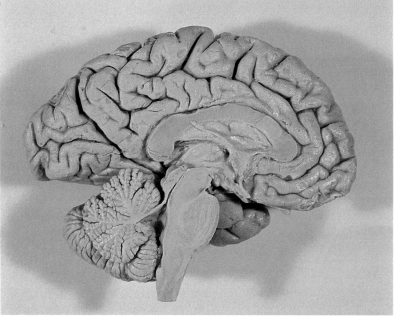

The determination of a person's right- or left-handedness is one trait which may eventually become controllable following future research with hormones. Isolation and manipulation of the main hormones responsible for handedness may predispose people towards "arts" or "sciences." Some researchers believe that left-handed individuals with right hemispheric dominance have tendencies toward musical and artistic abilities, whereas right-handed individuals with the left hemisphere (left) dominant tend to be better at languages and science.

For several years, scientists have researched the possibility of a hormonal method of contraception for men. Only future research will determine whether such a development is practical.

Beta-blocking drugs also inhibit the movement of sperm; exactly how is not yet known. Trials with beta-blockers in vaginal creams appear to be as effective as other "barrier" methods of contraception. Such a small amount of the drug is absorbed through the vaginal wall that there appears to be no systemic effect on the woman.

Problems of Infertility

Not being able to become pregnant can be a devastating problem for those maternal women who desperately want a family. Fortunately, an increased scientific understanding of reproduction, together with new medical technology, have led to sophisticated treatments that are now becoming available for infertility. These treatments of course depend on where the problem resides. If, for example, a woman's Fallopian tubes are blocked, the obstruction must be removed. If obstructed tubes cannot be repaired, ripe eggs may be gathered from the ovary, fertilized in a test tube and the tiny embryo put back into the womb.

Sometimes the problems are hormonal, and ripe eggs or sperm are not produced simply because the gonads are not receiving the correct hormone signals. Some women suffer from anovulatory menstrual cycles, so that menstruation occurs (often irregularly or at infrequent intervals), but an egg has not been released mid-cycle. Ovulation can be stimulated by giving an antiestrogen, which blocks the negative feedback action of ovarian estrogen, and so increases the secretion of gonadotropins. This may be sufficient to ensure the production of a ripe egg during the cycle.

The Uncertain Future

Major political and ethical problems are bound to be raised as hormone technology advances. Combine this with the ability to transfer genes to embryos, and the nightmare of Aldous Huxley's *Brave New World* looms near when the size, intellect and fertility of individuals can be controlled artificially.

Extra growth hormone genes have been transferred into mice along with a controlling gene that allows hormone production to increase. The result is that the mice grow larger than normal. Could such a technique be applied to humans to produce, say, a nation of basketball players? Would it be

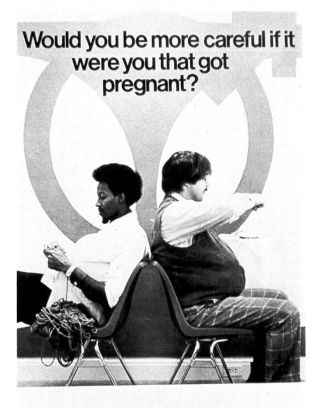

Would you be more careful if it were you that got pregnant?

possible to increase natural testosterone production by implanting the gene for the hormone which stimulates its production, before the child is born? This could produce superathletes at one end of the scale, or people with a high risk of coronary heart disease at the other.

A recent hypothesis suggests that higher levels of testosterone in the mother may affect the embryonic brain, making the right side dominant instead of the usual left hemisphere. As a result, the person is left-handed, but may have greater mathematical abilities. Unfortunately, such a person may be more likely to develop mental and allergic illness, especially if the exact balance is wrong.

Sometime soon, individual nations and the international community will have to begin making decisions about how far the hormonal or genetic manipulation of humankind should be allowed to progress. Even then, it may be easier to cheat than to detect cheating.

Glossary

acetylcholine a chemical that acts as a transmitter of signals at nerve ends.

ACTH adrenocorticotropic hormone.

Addison's disease a disease due to failure of the adrenal cortex to secrete hormones. Symptoms include wasting, weakness, low blood pressure and dark pigmentation of the skin.

adenoma a benign tumor in, or looking like, a gland.

adenosine triphosphate (ATP) a compound in which energy is stored in cells.

ADH antidiuretic hormone.

adrenal glands a pair of endocrine glands located just above the kidneys.

adrenocorticotropic hormone (ACTH) a hormone secreted by the pituitary which affects the function of the adrenal cortex. Also called adrenocorticotropin.

aldosterone a hormone from the adrenal cortex which affects sodium retention.

alpha cells cells in the islets of Langerhans of the pancreas that secrete glucagon.

α-MSH melanocyte-stimulating hormone.

anabolic steroids substances resembling hormones of the adrenal cortex and testes, which can produce large increases in muscle bulk.

androgens male sex hormones.

androsterone one of the androgens.

anemia lack of hemoglobin in the blood.

angiotensin a hormone producing a rise in blood pressure.

antibodies substances produced by an organism in response to foreign substances or organisms, which can neutralize these by binding to them.

antidiuretic hormone (ADH) a hormone of the hypothalamus, stored in the posterior pituitary, which causes reduced urine flow.

antireceptor agents chemicals that block a cell's response to a hormone by obstructing the hormone receptor sites.

ATP adenosine triphosphate.

autoregulation regulation of hormone production by direct effect of the hormone on the producing gland.

basal metabolic rate (BMR) the rate of energy production in the resting body.

beta cells cells in the islets of Langerhans of the pancreas that secrete insulin.

beta-blocker drugs stress-relieving drugs that block the action of epinephrine, reducing pulse rate, blood pressure and tremors.

bradykinin one of the hormones produced when blood plasma globulin is acted on by certain enzymes.

C cells cells in the thyroid gland that secrete calcitonin.

calcitonin a thyroid hormone that lowers the level of blood calcium.

catabolism the breaking down of body substance.

catecholamines a generic term for a group of hormonal substances including epinephrine, norepinephrine and dopamine.

cholecystokinin a duodenal hormone that makes the gall bladder contract.

cholesterol a fatty substance that is a precursor of steroid hormones.

chorionic gonadotropin a hormone released from the placental membranes that keeps the corpus luteum functional.

chromosomes the bodies within the cell nucleus that contain the genetic material in the form of DNA.

circadian rhythm a body rhythm, as of hormone secretion, which has a period of about 24 hours.

climacteric the period of physical and mental change associated with the natural cessation of menstruation in women and of active sexual participation by men.

colloid the viscid central part of thyroid follicles.

colon the large intestine.

colostrum the fluid produced from the breasts immediately after childbirth before the true milk, and high in proteins and antibodies.

Conn's syndrome excess production of steroid hormones affecting mineral balance, often caused by a small tumor of the adrenal glands.

corpus luteum the body formed from an ovarian follicle after an egg has been released.

cortex the outer layers of an organ such as a kidney or adrenal gland.

corticosterone an adrenal hormone.

Cushing's syndrome overproduction of steroid hormones by the adrenal glands.

cyclic adenosine 3′:5′-monophosphate (cAMP) an intracellular chemical believed to act as an intermediary to trigger the chain of events in the cell characteristic of some hormones (also known as cyclic AMP).

cytoplasmic receptors receptors within the cell to which hormones can attach.

diabetes insipidus a condition in which there is abnormally high urine production as a result of pituitary or brain dysfunction leading to lack of antidiuretic hormone.

diabetes mellitus a disease in which blood sugar and urine sugar are abnormally high.

DNA deoxyribonucleic acid, the chemical that carries the genetic code.

dopamine dihydroxyphenylalanine, an amino acid that has hormonal actions.

endocrine glands glands whose secretions are carried via the bloodstream (and not by a duct) to the point affected.

endometrium the internal layer of the uterus which is built up monthly to receive a fertilized ovum.

endorphins hormones found in the brain that appear to influence pain perception.

enteroglucagon a gut hormone that influences pancreatic secretion.

enkephalins hormones found in the brain that appear to influence pain perception.

enzymes proteins which mediate in chemical reactions within a body, like a catalyst facilitating the reaction, but not themselves consumed.

epinephrine a hormone secreted by the adrenal medulla and other sites in the body. Also known as adrenaline.

epithelial of the layer of tissue that covers or lines internal or external surfaces of the body.

erythropoietin a kidney hormone that stimulates production of red blood cells.

estrogen generic term for female sex hormones.

Fallopian tube the tube that carries an ovum from the ovary to the uterus.

feedback mechanism any mechanism, of machine or body, that is modified and regulated by its own products.

follicle-stimulating hormone (FSH) a hormone of the anterior pituitary that acts on the ovaries or on the testes.

follicle a small sac. The ovarian follicle contains the ripening ovum.

FSH follicle-stimulating hormone.

gastrin a hormone secreted by the stomach wall that stimulates acid secretion by the stomach.

genetic engineering artificial alteration of the genetic makeup of an organism.

GH growth hormone.

gigantism overgrowth due to excessive secretion of growth hormone by the pituitary gland.

glucagon a pancreatic hormone that stimulates breakdown of glycogen in

the liver and thus an increase in blood sugar.

glucocorticoids hormones secreted by the adrenal cortex that are important regulators of carbohydrate metabolism.

glucose a simple sugar which is transported in the bloodstream.

glycogen a carbohydrate storage product in cells, particularly those of the liver.

glycoprotein compounds of protein and carbohydrate, such as in mucus.

goiter enlargement of the thyroid gland caused by a disorder.

gonadotropins pituitary hormones that act on the reproductive glands.

Graafian follicle the sac in an ovary that surrounds the developing ovum.

growth hormone (GH) the growth-stimulating hormone secreted by the anterior pituitary.

growth hormone releasing factor a hormone from the hypothalamus that controls GH secretion from the pituitary.

Hashimoto's disease an autoimmune disease in which white blood cells attack the thyroid and cause goiter.

histamine a local hormone that dilates capillaries and makes them leaky, and plays a large part in allergic reactions.

hormone replacement therapy treatment of a disorder or of the effects of aging by the artificial provision of hormones.

hormones strictly, substances such as the secretions of the ductless glands that are produced at one place but have an effect on a distant organ. Sometimes used of substances with a more local effect.

human chorionic somatomammotropin a placental hormone that helps prepare the breasts to produce milk.

hydrocortisone cortisol, a steroid drug used to combat adrenal cortex insufficiency, and to treat arthritis and other inflammations.

hyper- a prefix meaning "over," used in compound words such as hyperthyroidism, meaning overactivity of the thyroid.

hypo- a prefix meaning "under," used in compound words such as hypothyroidism, meaning underactivity of the thyroid.

hypothalamus a cluster of cells at the base of the forebrain with a secretory function and important in the control of the endocrine system.

immunosuppressive drugs substances that suppress the normal reaction of the body to foreign substances or tissues.

insulin a hormone produced by the beta cells in the islets of Langerhans of the pancreas which facilitates entry of glucose into the body's cells.

interstitial describes the fluid-filled spaces between the cells of a tissue.

intrauterine within the womb, or uterus.

islets of Langerhans minute oval bodies of tissue within the pancreas where the hormones insulin and glucagon are made.

jaundice yellowing of the skin and eyes by bile pigments, symptomatic of a disorder.

kinases substances that transform precursor molecules into enzymes.

Klinefelter's syndrome a condition in which a man has an extra X chromosome in addition to the usual X and Y sex chromosomes.

lactation the production of milk.

lacteals lymphatic ducts in the intestine which carry a suspension of fats.

leukotrienes local hormones related to prostaglandins.

LH luteinizing hormone.

lipase an enzyme that breaks down fats.

luteinizing hormone a hormone of the anterior pituitary that stimulates ovulation and the formation of the corpus luteum.

luteolysis the breakdown of the corpus luteum.

lymphatic system a system of tubes (much like blood vessels) containing the colorless liquid lymph, which drains from the tissues.

lymphocytes small white corpuscles that occur in blood and lymph.

lymphoid tissue tissues connected with the lymph system.

medulla the central part of an organ such as a kidney or adrenal gland.

melanocyte-stimulating hormone (MSH) a hormone causing skin color changes in lower vertebrates, but of uncertain function in humans.

melatonin a pineal hormone influencing secretion of gonadotropins, and possibly of importance in controlling sleep.

metabolism the chemical changes taking place within organisms, whether building up or breaking down the tissues.

milk ejection reflex the hormone-mediated reflex of contraction of milk ducts in the breast in response to a baby's sucking.

mineral corticoids steroid hormones produced in the adrenal cortex which regulate mineral and fluid balance.

mucus the slimy, sticky fluid secreted by mucous glands.

myasthenia gravis an autoimmune disease in which the muscles are weakened.

myxedema a condition caused by thyroid deficiency, in which there is weight gain, slowing of metabolism and coarsening of the skin.

negative feedback regulation of a process by its own products, directly or indirectly, acting to stop or slow the process.

neural of, or connected with, nerves.

neuroendocrinology the study of the interrelationship of hormones and nerves.

neurohormones substances produced by nerves which can act as hormones.

neurohumoral produced by nerves, but acting via the bloodstream, as neurohormones.

neuron a nerve cell.

neurosecretory cells cells such as some in the pituitary gland with a nervous derivation but which secrete hormones.

norepinephrine a hormone produced in the adrenal medulla and also a transmitter at sympathetic nerve endings. It increases heart rate, increases muscle blood supply and releases glucose. Also called noradrenaline.

opioid peptides substances that mimic some of the painkilling effects of morphine, and which may also be important in controlling hormone secretion.

oral hypoglycemic agents substances which can be taken by mouth and which reduce blood sugar in some diabetics.

organotherapy treatment of disease by use of animal organs or their extracts.

osmoreceptors body receptors which can detect changes in the concentration of salts in the body fluids.

osteoarthritis disease of the joints in which the cartilage and bone degenerate.

ovulation the release of an ovum from the ovary.

oxytocin a hormone produced in the posterior pituitary. It stimulates contractions of the muscle of the uterus at childbirth and breast muscles to eject milk.

pancreas an organ containing digestive and endocrine glands whose secretions are effective in the first part of the small intestine.

pancreozymin a hormone of the small intestine that stimulates secretion of digestive enzymes from the pancreas.

parafollicular cells C cells of the thyroid.

parathormone hormone produced by the parathyroid glands, which raises calcium levels in the blood and assists in controlling calcium metabolism.

parathyroid glands four small bodies of endocrine tissue situated near the thyroid gland in the neck region.

peptides compounds of low molecular weight made up of amino acids.

pheochromocytoma a type of tumor in tissue derived from the adrenal medulla.

pineal gland a gland at the base of the brain, homologous with the third eye of some lower vertebrates. Its functions are poorly understood.

pituitary dwarf someone of small stature resulting from lack of growth hormone from the pituitary gland.

pituitary gland an endocrine gland below the brain and above the nasal cavity. Its hormones control the secretion of many of the other endocrine glands of the body.

placenta the structure formed by the fusion of outer embryonic membranes with the wall of the uterus by means of which substances are exchanged between the bloodstreams of the fetus and the mother.

plasma the liquid which bathes the body tissues; blood without the blood cells.

plasma membrane the membrane forming the outer boundary of the cytoplasm of the cell.

plasmid part of the genetic material of some bacteria; a bacterial chromosome.

posterior pituitary the rear lobe of the pituitary, derived from nervous tissue, and secreting ADH and oxytocin.

progesterone a hormone secreted by the corpus luteum that produces changes in the uterus which make it ready for pregnancy.

prohormones   inactive precursor molecules that can give rise to hormones.

prolactin   a hormone of the anterior pituitary that stimulates milk production.

prolactin-stimulating factor   a factor from the hypothalamus controlling pituitary secretion of prolactin.

prostacyclin   a type of prostaglandin that acts to prevent blood clotting.

prostaglandins   fatty acids that act as local hormones. They produce a wide variety of effects.

proteins   compounds of high molecular weight characteristic of living tissue and made up of amino acids.

pseudohermaphroditism   having the physical appearance of one sex but the genetic makeup and gonads of the other.

radiation therapy   the treatment of a diseased organ with penetrating radiation.

radioimmunoassay technique   a technique for using radioactive samples to trace small amounts of substances, such as hormones produced by the body.

renin   a hormone secreted by the kidney that helps to control blood pressure.

secretin   a hormone secreted by the small intestine which stimulates the secretion of pancreatic juices.

semen   the fluid secreted from the testes and their accessory glands and ejaculated at orgasm.

seminiferous tubules   the tubules within the testis in which sperm are made.

somatostatin   a hormone secreted by the hypothalamus that inhibits release of growth hormone from the pituitary.

somatotropin   growth hormone.

somatotropin-releasing factor   a hormone of the hypothalamus that promotes the release of growth hormone from the pituitary.

sphincter   a muscle which closes an orifice when contracted.

spleen   a blood-filled organ near the liver in which the blood cells are destroyed and lymphocytes are produced.

steroids   complex hydrocarbons which include hormones from the adrenal cortex and the gonads.

suprarenal glands   adrenal glands.

testicular feminization syndrome   a condition in which a genetic male fails to develop male characteristics in response to testosterone from the embryo testes, and has a female appearance.

testosterone   a male hormone produced by the testes.

thrombosis   the formation of a blood clot in a blood vessel.

thromboxane   a substance produced by blood platelets that enhances clotting.

thymus   an endocrine gland situated just behind the breastbone, important in the body's defense against disease.

thymusin   a thymus hormone that promotes the maturation of lymphocytes.

thyroglobulin   a protein-carbohydrate compound found in the colloid of the thyroid gland that is a precursor of thyroid hormones.

thyroid gland   an endocrine gland in the neck which has an important role in the control of energy metabolism.

thyroid-stimulating hormone   a hormone of the anterior pituitary that exerts control on secretion by the thyroid.

thyroiditis   inflammation of the thyroid.

thyrotoxicosis   disease caused by overactivity of the thyroid gland.

thyrotropin   thyroid-stimulating hormone.

thyrotropin-releasing hormone   a hormone secreted by the hypothalamus that stimulates the pituitary to release thyroid-stimulating hormone.

thyroxine (T_4)   a hormone produced by the thyroid gland which influences the body's metabolic rate.

transducers   devices or body organs that can receive input in one form of energy and output a different form.

trauma   a wound or injury.

triiodothyronine (T_3)   a hormone produced by the thyroid gland which influences the body's metabolic rate.

tuberculosis   a bacterial disease characterized by the formation of nodules in the body tissues.

Turner's syndrome   a condition in which a female has only one of the normal pair of X chromosomes.

uterus   the womb, the organ in which an embryo develops before birth.

vascular   pertaining to, or supplied with, vessels for the circulation of body fluids.

vasopressin   antidiuretic hormone.

vesicle   a small cavity or fluid-filled sac.

villi   one of the small processes lining the inside of the small intestine.

viruses   ultramicroscopic organisms capable of replicating themselves only within the cells of a host organism. Many cause diseases in humans.

von Recklinghausen's disease   a condition in which there is loss of calcium from bones due to overactivity of the parathyroid glands.

X chromosome   one of the sex chromosomes; females have two X chromosomes, males have only one.

xanthoma   a yellowish fibrous tumor occurring on the skin in some diseases.

Y chromosome   sex chromosome found only in males; the other of each pair is an X chromosome, as in females.

Illustration Credits

History of Hormones
8, *Medusa* by Lucien Levy/Palais de Tokyo, Paris/The Bridgeman Art Library. 10, Mary Evans Picture Library. 11, *The Rialto Bridge, Venice, from the north* by Canaletto/Christie's, London/The Bridgeman Art Library. 13, *The Four Humours* from *Barber Surgeons*/The British Museum/The Bridgeman Art Library. 14, Mary Evans Picture Library. 15, Mary Evans Picture Library. 16, Biophoto Associates. 17, The British Library. 18, Ann Ronan Picture Library. 19, *Poultry* by William Huggins/The Bridgeman Art Library. 20, Ann Ronan Picture Library. 21, The Mansell Collection. 22a, The Mansell Collection. 22b, Gene Cox. 23, *Praying Hands* by Albrecht Dürer/Albertina, Vienna/The Bridgeman Art Library. 25, David Parker/Science Photo Library.

The Organic Orchestra
26, *The Wet Nurse* by Alfred Roll/Musée des Beaux Arts, Lille/The Bridgeman Art Library. 28, Alexander Tsiaras/Science Photo Library. 29, Science Photo Library. 30, Science Photo Library. 31, From the Romance of Amir Hamza/Victoria and Albert Museum/The Bridgeman Art Library. 32, **Mick Gillah**. 33, Sally and Richard Greenhill. 34a, Professor T Blundell/Science Photo Library. 34b, Martin Dohrn/Science Photo Library. 35a, John Topham Photo Library. 35b, John Topham Photo Library. 35c, BBC Hulton Picture Library. 36, Hank Morgan/Science Photo Library. 37, *Heroes Recruiting at Kelsey's* by James Gillray/Private Collection/The Bridgeman Art Library. 38, Biophoto Associates. 39, Jan Hinsch/Science Photo Library. 40, Science Source/Science Photo Library. 41, Mick Rock/Camerapix Hutchison. 43, *Portrait of Sabartes* by Pablo Picasso/Pushkin Fine Arts Museum/The Bridgeman Art Library. 44, Anthony Blake. 45, The Photosource. 46, Biophoto Associates. 47, *Melencolia* by Albrecht Dürer/Guildhall Library, City of London/The Bridgeman Art Library. 48, Biophoto Associates. Foldout, (outside A) Mary Evans Picture Library, (outside B) Biophoto Associates, (inside) **Mick Saunders, Shirley Willis**, (outside C) John Watney, (outside D) Mary Evans Picture Library. 49, Neville Presho/Zefa UK Ltd. 50, **Mick Gillah**. 51, David Parker/Science Photo Library. 52, Biophoto Associates. 53, *Mexican Shawl* by Percy Wyndham Lewis/City of Bristol Museum and Art Gallery/The Bridgeman Art Library.

The Chemical Conductor
56, Patrick Lynch/Science Photo Library.

58a, **Aziz Khan**. 58b, Ann Ronan Picture Library. 59, John Bannister delivering a lecture/University of Glasgow/The Bridgeman Art Library. 60, Yale University Art Gallery, Gift of Mrs Cushing. 61, *"I am half sick of shadows"* said the Lady of Shallott by S H Meteyard/The Bridgeman Art Library. 62, Ivan Polunin/Natural History Photographic Agency. 63, **Aziz Khan**. 64, Dr Gerald Schatten/Science Photo Library. 65a, Zefa UK Ltd. 65b, Ann Ronan Picture Library. 66, C James Webb. 67a, Heather Angel/Biofotos. 67b, Sally and Richard Greenhill. 68, **Aziz Khan**. 69, Peter Johnson/Natural History Photographic Agency. 70, St Bartholomew's Hospital, London. 71, *Las Meninas* by Velasquez/Prado, Madrid/The Bridgeman Art Library. 72, Sally and Richard Greenhill. 73, *Jack and the Beanstalk* by Walter Crane/Victoria and Albert Museum/The Bridgeman Art Library. 74, Ann Ronan Picture Library. 75a, *Execution of the Defenders of Madrid* by Francisco Goya/Prado, Madrid/The Bridgeman Art Library. 75b, Gene Cox.

Hormonal Harmony
76, *The train at night* by Lionel Walden/Gavin Graham Gallery/The Bridgeman Art Library. 78, *Flying Mercury* by Giambologna/Louvre, Paris/The Bridgeman Art Library. 79a, *Waterloo* by G Newton/Cheltenham Art Gallery/The Bridgeman Art Library. 79b, Astrid Kage/Science Photo Library. 80a, **Aziz Khan**. 80b, **Aziz Khan**. 81, Kobal Collection. 82a, Ford Motor Company. 82b, Tony Stone Associates. 83, National Westminster Bank. 84, Photoresources. 85, **Mick Gillah**. 86, **Aziz Khan**. 87, *The Colossus* by Francisco Goya/Prado, Madrid/The Bridgeman Art Library. 88a, Robin Williams/Science Photo Library. 88b, Robin Williams/Science Photo Library. 89, Tony Stone Associates. 90, Dr Roland King/Science Photo Library. 91a, C James Webb. 91b, Dr Tony Brain/Science Photo Library. 92, Amersham International. 93, Amersham International.

Balancing the System
94, *Autumn* by Guiseppe Arcimboldo/Brescia Pincoteca, Scala. 96a **Aziz Khan**. 96b, Ann Ronan Picture Library. 97, Anthony Blake. 98, **Mick Saunders**. 99a, Biophoto Associates. 99b, Gene Cox. 100, Erik Leigh Simmons/Imagebank. 101, National Railway Museum, York. 102, Gene Cox. 103, *The Feast*, from Peter Pan/Private Collection/The Bridgeman Art Library. 104, John Egan/Camerapix Hutchison. 105a,

J F Gennaro/Science Photo Library. 105b, British Steel. 106a, Anthony Blake. 106b, Biophoto Associates. 107, J Behnke/Zefa UK Ltd. 108, **Aziz Khan**. 109a, Kobal Collection. 109b, Camerapix Hutchison.

Chemistry of Creation
110, From the *Akbar Nama*/Victoria and Albert Museum/The Bridgeman Art Library. 112, Michael Abbey/Science Photo Library. 113, Teasy/Zefa UK Ltd. 114, **Mick Gillah**. 115, Zefa UK Ltd. 116, Tony Stone Associates. 117a Tony Stone Associates. 117b, Mary Evans Picture Library. 118, *An Apartment in the Harem of Sheikh Sadat* by Frank Dillon/Victoria and Albert Museum/The Bridgeman Art Library. 119, **Mick Gillah**. 120a, Manfred Kage/Science Photo Library. 120b, C James Webb. 121, *The Moon* by Kunisada/The British Museum/The Bridgeman Art Library. 122, Robin Williams/Science Photo Library. 123, IPPF/FPA Hong Kong. 124, Martin Dohrn/Science Photo Library. 125, David Parker/Science Photo Library. 126a, **Mick Gillah**. 126b, Sally and Richard Greenhill. 128, **Mick Gillah**. 129, *The Novice* by Alfred Elmore/Bury Art Gallery/The Bridgeman Art Library.

Fiction or Future
130, Adrian Murrell/Allsport. 132, Mary Evans Picture Library. 133, *A Leicester Sow* by W H Davis/Dr C I Davenport Jones/The Bridgeman Art Library. 134, Barnaby's Picture Library. 135, *The Children in the Wood* by James Sant/Roy Miles Gallery/The Bridgeman Art Library. 136, Sally and Richard Greenhill. 137, John Topham Picture Library. 138a, **Mick Saunders**. 138b, Biophoto Associates. 139, Martin Dohrn/Science Photo Library. 140, **Mick Saunders**. 141, Sally and Richard Greenhill. 142a, Tony Stone Associates. 142b, Zefa UK Ltd. 143, Camerapix Hutchison. 144a, **Mick Saunders**. 144b, **Mick Saunders**. 145, **Mick Saunders**. 146a, S Stammers/Science Photo Library. 146b, C James Webb. 147, John Topham Picture Library. 148a, Sally and Richard Greenhill. 148b, Biophoto Associates. 149, IPPF.

Index